RETURN ON HUMAN EXPERIENCE

Eight Principles to Inspire Excellence in Healthcare

JASON A. WOLF, PHD, CPXP
STACY PALMER, CPXP

Return on Human Experience: Eight Principles to Inspire Excellence in Healthcare

987654321
First Edition
Printed in the United States of America.

Cover design by Jake Clark, Pithy Wordsmithery
Interior layout by Dave Vasudevan, Pithy Wordsmithery
Copy editing by Nils Kuehn, Pithy Wordsmithery
Proofreading by Scott Morrow and Katharine Dvorak, Pithy Wordsmithery

ISBN: 979-8-9902272-3-1 (Paperback)
ISBN: 979-8-9902272-4-8 (Ebook)
ISBN: 979-8-9902272-5-5 (Hardback)

Jason A. Wolf
jason.wolf@theberylinstitute.org
www.theberylinstitute.org

Stacy Palmer
stacy.palmer@theberylinstitute.org
www.theberylinstitute.org

Library of Congress Control Number: 2024916405

What People Are Saying...

"I'm awestruck by Jason Wolf and Stacy Palmer and their groundbreaking book on achieving 'experience excellence' in healthcare. With inspiring vision, perseverance, and community-building expertise, they have built a worldwide movement, engaging thousands of healthcare professionals worldwide in building an entirely NEW and comprehensive body of knowledge about how to rethink and elevate the human experience in healthcare for the sake of patients, families, communities, and everyone engaged in healthcare work. This wonderful, easy-to-read book describes the state of the science and the state of the art, so everyone who wants to improve the human experience in healthcare has a playbook for achieving breakthroughs in their organizations."

Wendy Leebov
Author and activist for transforming the patient experience
Founder, Language of Caring

"*Return on Human Experience* is a compelling recognition of the real value and return on investment for committing to the human experience in healthcare. Through the collaboration of contributions, insights, and the lived experience of The Beryl Institute's diverse global community, Jason Wolf and Stacy Palmer have authored a unique and leading-edge body of work. This truly is a must-read for what works in the transformation of the human experience in healthcare."

Tony Serge
Senior executive, patient and family advisor
Co-chair and past co-chair of patient and family advisor boards

"In embracing the needs and perspectives of everybody from the patient to the caregiver, from the workforce to the community, *Return on Human Experience* reveals a compelling blueprint for a true healthcare movement and raises the rallying cry for a broader, inclusive commitment to the human experience."

Dennis W. Pullin, FACHE
President and CEO, Virtua Health

"Over the last 15 years, The Beryl Institute has played a pivotal role in building the field of patient experience, creating standards and a community of practice that are now recognized as the gold standard across the healthcare industry. This book is a phenomenal compendium of the framework and principles that have taken us from a tactical focus on 'patient experience' to a visionary understanding of 'human experience.' I strongly recommend *Return on Human Experience* as a phenomenal go-to resource for any leader who wants to understand and transform the experience for all within their organization."

Rick Evans
SVP and chief experience officer, New York-Presbyterian Hospital

"*Return on Human Experience* should be the go-to book for all leaders as they strive to fulfill the mission of their organization. Its guiding principles are actions that profoundly move us closer to creating an excellence experience for our communities in healthcare. The book shares encounters of learning, growing, and collaboration and clearly defines these guiding principles for us all. Thank you for giving us this gift to share with others and to keep us on the journey to better the human experience. As stated in this book, 'There is a true return on an investment in human experience.'"

Cheryl Call, CAVS
Manager—volunteer, chaplaincy, hospitality, and gift shop services
Intermountain Health | Utah Valley Hospital

"As a patient who lives with my conditions 24/7, *Return on Human Experience* gives me hope. Hope for systems that will continue to strive to work with those receiving and providing care and the communities they live in, to drive impact and value through what matters most, to create meaningful connections and to improve outcomes."

Claire Snyman
Healthcare advocate and patient experience consultant

"Just like The Beryl Institute itself, *Return on Human Experience* is an invaluable resource to healthcare professionals committed to building and sustaining a culture of compassion and empathy in their organizations and their community. After more than 40 years in this business, I have gained so much knowledge and inspiration through the Institute and the guiding principles outlined in this book."

Carol Santalucia
Healthcare consultant and champion for healthcare experience
Former director of service excellence, Cleveland Clinic

"As a volunteer leader, I believe that The Beryl Institute community provides important insight by sharing their personal perceptions about the care they deliver and have received. In turn, their voices become an important part in guiding change. *Return on Human Experience* helps organizations understand just how important *all* voices are to the human experience."

Beth Daddario, CAVS
Director, volunteers and guest services, Inspira Health

"Patient experience has long been an intangible aspect of healthcare, but *Return on Human Experience* gives it shape and form. It reveals that experience is as crucial, if not more so, than the numbers we often chase. It is a true playbook on human experience. I get goosebumps reading this book."

Joyce K. Nazario, CPXP
Patient experience excellence head, Metro Pacific Health

"The Beryl Institute is the greatest example of how to connect people through a common purpose and mobilize a global community to share knowledge. *Return on Human Experience* translates a journey of learning and collective growth that will help you to put in practice the core principles of people-centered care and human experience in healthcare."

Marcelo Alvarenga, MD, MSc, CPXP
CEO, ConectaExp
Co-founder and president, SOBREXP | Brazilian Society of Patient Experience and Person-Centered Care

"Thank you to Jason Wolf and Stacy Palmer for critically explaining the value of human caring in healthcare for our patients and families, our healthcare professionals, and the communities we serve. *Return on Human Experience* is the prescription we all need to guide our experience strategies and to achieve success."

Alexie Puran, MD, MS, FACEP, FAAP, CPXP

Pediatric emergency medicine physician, NYC Health + Hospitals/Harlem
Assistant professor of clinical pediatrics, Columbia University

"*Return on Human Experience* shows how the idea of human beings caring for human beings helps create a healthcare world where everyone belongs, is respected, and receives excellent care. It reinforces that accountability creates trust, teamwork leads to quality, and our humanity must rest at the heart of healthcare."

Rosie Bartel
Patient advisor

"*Return on Human Experience* is a beacon of hope and inspiration for all in healthcare. This book brilliantly captures the essence of what it means to create environments where every interaction exudes compassion and every moment feels deeply personal. A must-read for anyone committed to transforming healthcare, it showcases a global community's collective wisdom and unwavering dedication to fostering a culture of genuine care and healing."

Anne Marie Hadley
Chief experience officer, NSW Health

"*Return on Human Experience* shares the importance of improving the human experience while navigating the complex and evolving factors impacting these efforts. It outlines the critical culture and work necessary to lead impactful change in healthcare around the world."

Kim Pedersen
Director, operations, patient support services, Marianjoy Rehabilitation Hospital | Northwestern Medicine

"Patient experience is a critical tool in today's healthcare experience, and it's one that provides lasting benefits. *Return on Human Experience* provides ways to invest in your organization's efforts to ensure an exceptional experience for the patients, families, and caregivers you serve."

Alex Seblatnigg, CAVS, CPXP
Director of volunteer services and internal engagement, Shepherd Center

"An invaluable resource for anyone committed to enhancing patient care, *Return on Human Experience* captures the essence of what it means to truly understand and improve the patient experience. Through insightful research and case studies, it offers practical strategies aligned with The Beryl Institute's eight principles to guide experience excellence, ensuring a holistic approach to patient care. A must-read for healthcare professionals dedicated to making a meaningful impact."

Alpa Vyas
Senior vice president, chief patient experience and operational performance officer, Stanford Health Care

"Transforming healthcare starts with a commitment to human experience. *Return on Human Experience* provides a road map for healthcare leaders, practitioners, and anyone seeking to create a more equitable and patient-centered system. The practical framework presented emphasizes the power of a strong organizational culture, dedicated leadership, and a deep commitment to health equity. By actively engaging patients, families, and the community, we can build a healthcare system that truly serves everyone."

Alina Moran, MPA, FACHE, FABC
President, Dignity Health—California Hospital Medical Center

"Finding your way through the valley of human experience in healthcare will be much easier with this book. It gathers core principles, powerful illustrations, and wise advice. If you are committed to bringing human experience in healthcare to the next level, you'll find not only why it is important but also how you can achieve it. This book is indispensable!"

Amah Kouevi
CEO, French Patient Experience Institute

Dedication

To Tiffany Christensen.

An unparalleled voice for what all healthcare could do to be better each day, who provided us with new lenses through which to see, an appreciation for all that was possible, and a call to move forward with purpose.

You are forever missed.

Contents

Foreword

Michael Dowling and Sven Gierlinger

This book arrives at a pivotal moment for healthcare. We stand at a crossroads where the imperative to deliver exceptional clinical care intersects with the equally vital need to nurture the human beings at the heart of every interaction. This is the essence of *Return on Human Experience: Eight Principles to Inspire Excellence in Healthcare*, a timely and essential guide for transforming healthcare from the inside out.

The authors, Jason A. Wolf and Stacy Palmer, pioneers in the field of healthcare experience, invite us on a journey that began with a simple yet profound realization: healthcare is about "human beings caring for human beings." This understanding, woven throughout these pages, transcends the traditional, transactional, siloed view of healthcare, urging us to embrace a more holistic perspective—one that celebrates the human spirit with dignity and respect.

To care for others—to commit to selflessness, to walk alongside patients and family caregivers through life's most monumental and poignant moments—is a privilege. This distinction is what makes healthcare stand apart from other industries. The work that healthcare leaders, providers, and professionals do each day is inspiring because of this complexity. There is no greater honor.

This book eloquently captures the evolution of the patient experience movement. It serves as encouragement and validation that this pursuit is meaningful and necessary for where we are in society today. Human experience has become mission critical, moving beyond the confines of satisfaction surveys and clinical outcomes, delving into the intricate interplay between patients, families, care partners, the workforce, and the communities they serve. The themes of partnership and collaboration further underscore the intersectionality of engagement, safety, and experience and that everything is connected. Through compelling real-world examples and actionable insights, the authors illuminate the eight guiding principles that form the bedrock of experience excellence. These principles are not mere theoretical constructs; they are practical tools for building a culture of trust, empathy, humanism, and transformation. Regardless of where your organization is in its human experience journey, these principles will help guide sustainable change across diverse care environments.

Return on Human Experience makes a compelling case for the tangible value of investing in human experience. It demonstrates how prioritizing the well-being of the workforce translates into improved patient care, how fostering genuine partnerships with patients and family caregivers leads to better outcomes, and how embracing a commitment to health equity uplifts entire communities.

This book is more than a guide; it is a call to action. It challenges us to move beyond incremental improvements and embrace a bold vision for the future of healthcare—one where human connection is the driving force behind every decision, every interaction, and every outcome. Collectively, we must continue to challenge the status quo and bring forth innovative ideas. In reflecting on how far we have come in our pursuit of human-centered care, the time is now to focus on designing and delivering a brighter, more human-centered tomorrow.

Where healthcare goes next is in our hands. We invite you to join us on this exciting journey of transformation. Now more than ever, humans need compassion, connection, inclusion, and grace. Fueled by optimism and grounded in professional purpose, let us be reminded of the impact that one person can have on another's life. May the stories, insights, and exemplars within these pages inspire you to become a champion for human experience in your own sphere of influence. Together, we can create a healthcare system that truly honors the humanity of those who deliver care and those who receive it.

Michael Dowling, president and CEO
Sven Gierlinger, senior vice president, chief experience officer
Northwell Health

Foreword

Dr. Airica Steed, EdD, RN, MBA, FACHE

There was once a successful healthcare executive who made sure to always carve time out of her evenings to play with her young daughter.

One evening, the executive was busy with an important project for work. She would not be able to spend time with her daughter, yet she wanted to give her something to keep busy.

The executive looked around her office and spotted an industry magazine with a full-page advertisement on the back cover. The ad showed a large, colorful map of the world.

This gave her an idea. She grabbed her scissors, cut the page from the magazine, and then carefully tore the page into dozens of tiny pieces.

The executive walked into her daughter's bedroom and explained that because she had a bit of extra work to do, she could not spend time with her just now. She led the girl to the kitchen table, gave her a roll of tape, and spread the torn pieces of paper across the table.

"This is a puzzle of our world," the executive said. "It is a mess right now, and it needs to be put back together. Can you help me?"

"Of course, Mommy," the girl replied.

"After you are finished, we can play," said the executive, knowing full well that it would take hours for the girl to fit and tape the pieces together.

But only 15 minutes later, just as the executive had gotten absorbed in a spreadsheet, the girl walked in holding up a perfectly taped-together page.

"I'm done, Mommy. Let's play."

The executive was stunned.

"My goodness! How did you do that?!"

"It was hard at first," the daughter said, "but then I figured out that on the back of the picture of the world was a picture of a person. Then it was simple. I put the person together, and the whole world fell into place."

I am not sure where I first heard this story, but as I read an early draft of the landmark book you now hold in your hands, I was reminded of the powerful message of this parable: the world comes together not when we focus on the pieces—the spreadsheets, the slide decks, the silos—but when we focus on the people, the humanity.

"Patient experience" has been at the center of my work at every position I have been blessed to hold in my career. It has been my life's work. I was called to it by my mother, the most brilliant, gifted, intelligent, and hardworking person I have ever known.

Until she got sick in her early 40s, she was a strong and successful nurse, striding the hospital halls during her shifts, lifting and inspiring everyone who encountered her. At first, her symptoms weren't serious. Cancer was the furthest thing from our minds.

But she got sicker. She was misdiagnosed, again and again and again. Over just 18 months, my mother deteriorated from a model of physical health to a mere shell of herself: blind, deaf, disabled, and often incoherent. She died not from the rare form of leukemia she had but from the side effects of the experimental treatment she received—treatment our family was never informed about and that my mother would have never consented to had she been in her right mind when asked to sign the form.

In just my early 20s, I had a front-row seat to some of the worst "misses" of America's broken healthcare system: mistakes, misdiagnosis, mistreatment, and miscommunication. I watched as my mother and my family were misled, dismissed, and ignored by the very people charged to heal and help us. Instead of delivering dignity, they delivered despair.

For my mother and my family—as with far too many people of color—"patient experience" was a tragedy.

I vowed to myself back then that I would devote my career to making sure other families did not endure such needless suffering and heartbreak.

Since then, my mother has become my guardian angel. She is with me every day, guiding me. She's next to me in every meeting, at my side during every rounding, and in the audience at every speech and presentation.

She helps make sure that I am always keeping the important things—patient experience, health equity, and humanity—top of mind.

I believe I am far from alone. I believe that countless former patients, family members, and caregivers occupy the subconscious spirits and guide the righteous work of the many great minds and talents working to improve the patient experience, increase access, and eliminate health disparities.

Stacy Palmer and Jason Wolf have done something miraculous in these pages.

They have taken a subject near and dear—*and inside*—my heart and enlarged it, widened it, lengthened it, and deepened it until it has become its absolute right size.

Patient experience is *human experience*.

And by "human," Stacy and Jason include not just patients, family members, loved ones, care partners, and friends; they include the caregivers, the entire workforce, the complete continuum of care, and, yes, the entire community. They do it because each of them is a vital part of any organization's human experience.

Not only have Stacy and Jason—and The Beryl Institute and its partners—boldly broadened the definition of experience, but they have crafted this transformative text that will allow all of us to achieve an entirely new dimension of hope, healing, and health for our patients, our caregivers, and our community.

This is not just an elevation of a concept; it is a program of action to achieve it.

Perhaps the best news: when we apply their elegant distillations—outlined in the guiding principles, the Experience Framework, the "Declaration for Human Experience"— we will see positive, measurable impacts in virtually every area of our organizations, from outcomes to operations, from reputation in the community to wellness in the community, from efficiency to equity.

Over their 15 years of work and collaboration, Stacy and Jason have taken all the pieces of the puzzle of patient experience and put together a blueprint to achieve perhaps everything we strive for in healthcare.

How did they do it?

By putting humanity first, the world just fell into place.

Dr. Airica Steed, EdD, RN, MBA, FACHE
Healthcare executive
Cleveland, Ohio

Preface

This book marks a critical milestone in the journey of The Beryl Institute and what led me to tackle this work with such passion. Catalyzed by my own experience in healthcare leadership, where I saw collaboration give way to competition and the sharing of ideas as antithetical to competitive success, I realized, or at least hoped, that there was a better way. I was confident that if we could build a space where collaboration and community were foundational, and the purpose was not solely about how each organization performed but rather how transformation occurred, we had an opportunity to bend the arc of healthcare.

The people who chose to come into this space — The Beryl Institute community space — did not heed a call to follow an idea. Rather, they stepped higher into their own purpose in a commitment to something greater. For almost 15 years now, we have grown and engaged leaders around the world who believe in the idea that what they give in ideas and lessons learned they get back tenfold — that this opportunity for exponential and shared improvement could be practically helpful and profoundly inspirational. I believe that this book honors that very idea, as its pages reflect both the practical and inspirational.

Now is the time to share this story. And there is no better partner to co-author it with than my colleague and friend Stacy Palmer, who helped turn so much of what was once vision and hope into structure and possibility. Stacy's leadership in our movement has been a solid backbone for all we have achieved together as a community. The story we share on these pages reflects how we, as leaders, have helped to weave the power of our community in tangible practice into a true return on value for all who invest in and commit to transforming human experience. I know that our community has shifted the direction of healthcare, however subtly or significantly, forever. And for that, I am eternally grateful.

—Jason A. Wolf

In 2010, I was presented with an incredible opportunity to help build The Beryl Institute as a membership community. It is an ongoing adventure that will always be a highlight of my career. Early on, I knew we were creating something special and impactful—but I don't believe I grasped how transformational this journey would be. How could I? From the intricacies of growing a compassionate team, fostering a vast library of resources, and encouraging meaningful connections, every step along the way has been intentional and essential. We have been honored to build both a professional home for a growing field of leaders and a business case for why this work is so critical to the evolution of healthcare.

Without a doubt, the best part has been the many individuals we have met along the way who have committed their time, energy, and experience to help shape this community. I admire and adore the passion of our members at The Beryl Institute to make a lasting impact. Experience leaders are committed to driving improvements by changing the conversation in healthcare—but it's not always easy. We often hear how they feel alone in this work, prompting one of our goals to eliminate that isolation through this community.

My goal with this book is that it will serve as another connecting force—a lifeline that the healthcare community needs—as it offers insights and tactics to keep these individuals moving forward on their respective journeys. Even more importantly, I believe it will help build a support system around them with allies who will be instrumental in bringing their vision to life. My hope is that senior leaders entrusted to guide healthcare organizations will take the messages that lie within these pages as inspiration to transform their organizations to places of great compassion, respect, and collaboration.

I am beyond grateful to Jason Wolf for leading The Beryl Institute, and the experience movement, with his incredible mission, vision, and commitment. And I especially thank him for the invitation to be his partner in this endeavor.

—Stacy Palmer

Introduction

Imagine a healthcare facility where every interaction feels seamless, every individual expresses compassion, and every exchange is deeply personal. Imagine that from the moment you step through the doors, you feel a sense of relief and confidence, understanding that you are in a place dedicated not just to treating ailments but to nurturing health, well-being, and healing in a comprehensive way.

Imagine, if you could.

Imagine walking out of that facility and sharing those feelings and observations with family, friends, and others in your community. Imagine hearing stories about a healthcare facility that evoked those feelings in someone else when it's time to make your own healthcare decisions.

Imagine the difference it would make in so many ways.

What we've described above isn't wishful thinking. It is already a reality in many healthcare organizations around the world—and it is an expressed objective for many others. As professionals who are passionate about transforming human experience in healthcare, we have come together in this book to reinforce our shared commitment and reaffirm our shared purpose. This commitment and purpose were brought to life through our work of building and growing The Beryl Institute community. And through that work, we have served as a catalyst for connection and collaboration around experience excellence, informed and inspired by the sharing of information, resources, stories, and lessons learned from members of our global community.

We believe that what we have built together as a community is unique. And it is that uniqueness that is reflected on the pages that follow. This book brings together and reflects on the contributions, insights, and experience of a diverse and robust global community that has learned, shared, and grown together for nearly 15 years. This sense of collaborative effort and commitment to one another in the purpose of something better for all in healthcare is a powerful statement of all that we and The Beryl Institute community have stood—and continue to stand—for. This was our commitment 15 years ago, remains our commitment today, and will continue to be our commitment for years to come.

A SPIRIT OF GENEROSITY

Since the inception of The Beryl Institute, we've understood that in order to shine a light on the true value of a commitment to experience in healthcare, we need others who can help kindle that light. To that end, we remain dedicated to building a global network of purposeful professionals, practitioners, innovators, patients, family members,

Since the inception of The Beryl Institute, we've understood that in order to shine a light on the true value of a commitment to experience in healthcare, we need others who can help kindle that light.

and care partners. Through a belief in "sharing wildly and borrowing willingly," that network has solidified a community that has helped build a foundation for experience excellence in healthcare. That foundation—grounded in a core definition, pushed forward by guiding principles, expanded through an integrated framework, and advanced through a commitment to human experience—reflects a reality that has a positive and extensive impact on healthcare outcomes overall.

As we reflect on the stories we've heard and the practices we've seen along our journey, we continue to recognize the pivotal role this community has played, and continues to play, in shaping and reaffirming our work. In fostering a space where people generously and openly share both their struggles and successes, we have encountered a broad range of situations, each one offering valuable lessons and insights. Numerous healthcare organizations have selflessly welcomed us in and actively engaged in sharing their stories and accomplishments, their challenges and innovations—the common motivation being that when we share the lessons we've learned in order to help others, we are granted greater opportunities ourselves to learn and improve together.

Through this community, we have had the extraordinary privilege not only to observe but also to actively participate in shaping the landscape of the healthcare experience. We have also been in the fortunate position to serve as a reflection of the experiences of this incredibly generous community. The success of our movement, the growth of our community, and the lessons we share on the pages that follow are grounded in this unwavering spirit of generosity.

A COMMITMENT TO COMMUNITY

Clearly, community is at the heart of our work—and it's no coincidence to us that the word "community" includes "unity." Once again, this reflects our commitment to unite those in healthcare together around shared beliefs, values, and best practices to improve the healthcare experience. All that we do is built on this sense of collaboration.

This is how we have worked to shape and establish the field of healthcare experience. Through collaboration, we've built a community, a formal body of knowledge, and a collective understanding established through research and vast experience. These resources provide a means to codify, digest, access, and share information that supports everyone on their own experience journey.

We started with a simple idea: to establish a definition and framework through which we could individually, organizationally, and collectively understand where we are, identify the opportunities at hand, and then connect to the resources and solutions that will help us continue down the road to experience excellence. Today, this notion has morphed into much more.

Given that our experience and reflections now traverse a decade and a half, we would be remiss not to acknowledge that some of the examples discussed on the following pages may no longer be in practice as originally shared, and in some instances, even the organizations noted may no longer exist. However, we strongly believe—and it is important that we emphasize here—that the relevance of these examples lies not in their current practice but in their lasting impact and the learning and improvement they've inspired. Their continued prominence as critical practice, despite the passage of time and number of them we have seen, speaks volumes about their efficacy. Simply, we have seen what works.

It is also through the extensive collaboration and co-creation within our community that the work itself has evolved. Healthcare has and always will be about human beings caring for human beings. Yet we risk losing touch with this fundamental principle when we add layers of professional titles, technical skills, processes, protocols, and diagnostic labels. For healthcare to be effective and meet the needs of those it serves, of those who choose caring for others as a profession, and of those in the community, this principle—that collaboration and shared learning are the foundation of expanding improvement and excellence—must remain at the heart of every intention and action.

AN EXPANDED CONVERSATION ON HUMAN EXPERIENCE

We believed early on that an integrated approach would be essential to build the institute's community. A true and comprehensive commitment to experience must be inclusive of caring for not only those we serve in healthcare but also those who show up to serve every day and the communities in which our healthcare organizations operate. This evolution from improving patient experience to transforming human experience was based on the premise that it was time to rethink the traditional dialogue on healthcare experience that often centered solely on patient interactions within clinical settings.

A comprehensive approach recognizes both the influence of the workforce and the broader societal and systemic factors that impact healthcare. By adopting a more expansive lens, we can address these multifaceted dimensions of experience that extend beyond the confines of traditional clinical settings. With this perspective, we can also help avoid the potential complacency of simply applying tactics to problems. Experience is much more than that—it is both a foundational and strategic imperative for healthcare overall.

By including both the workforce and community, we build meaningful partnerships with, and engagement of, those who work in healthcare and those in thriving and healthier communities. With less emphasis on tactics, on the "what to do," and more emphasis on true experience, on how organizations choose "to be," we move from checklist-driven actions to a comprehensive and strategic effort. It is the "why this is so important" and the "how we get there," grounded in collaboration and community and framed by an integrated approach, that provides both the inspiration and framing for this book.

WHY THIS BOOK AND WHAT TO EXPECT

The framing this book proposes is designed to do exactly that—to thoughtfully push us forward, to nudge us gently through discomfort in a shared willingness to address something bigger with a new approach. Its commitment is to share why this is important as well as to address how to get there through examples we have been privileged to encounter over the years. Ultimately, this book makes the case that there is real value in a commitment to this work. There is a true return on an investment in human experience.

On the following pages, we broaden our focus beyond the real and critical needs of individuals and patients to encompass this holistic view of the entire continuum of care, including leadership, the healthcare workforce, organizational culture, patients, family members and care partners, the interactions we allow, and the equity and access we ensure. This approach is based on the intricate interplay between these elements, linked across the entire patient journey—from well before someone enters a clinical space to long after they leave.

The chapters that follow are interconnected as important pieces of an essential whole. Reading them in isolation, similar to looking at experience from distinct organizational or operational silos, risks missing their critical interplay—where they weave together and how they build upon each other. The chapters should be read with the understanding that they collectively contribute to ensuring experience excellence overall.

Chapters 2 through 9 are anchored by one of our eight guiding principles, each representing an action that is essential to a comprehensive experience strategy. We believe that these principles are the foundational building blocks to organizational effectiveness and a means to achieving sustained outcomes for any organization's commitment to experience excellence, which is why they also serve as a road map for this book. It is our hope that the guiding principles are aspirational and affirmative statements about where we, as individuals and organizations, stand collectively and where we, as the human experience movement, should focus our efforts going forward.

These core chapters also each begin with three key takeaways—crucial insights that encapsulate the essence of each topic. Whether you delve into each chapter in its entirely or simply absorb these key points, you will undoubtedly gain valuable knowledge and inspiration. The content within each chapter then includes broad conceptual buckets with examples that signify the primary concepts we have discovered and curated through our community in growing the institute. The chapters conclude by highlighting the impact that each of these foundational principles can help organizations realize, emphasizing the tangible benefits that arise from prioritizing human experience in healthcare.

We feel honored to be building a global community that is so committed and passionate about transforming human experience in healthcare. We remain inspired by all the many contributions—shared through lessons learned, proven practices, and successes and misses—that have been made in this commitment to something bigger.

This is why, as leaders of The Beryl Institute, we believe the time for a book that frames experience in this new, practical, and strategically applicable way is now—a book that acknowledges what works, gives guidance to those who seek it, and offers encouragement to those who need it. This idea of generosity and connection, shared learning and support, has always been central to all we have done in our work. Our sincerest hope is that you feel that purpose on the pages that follow.

If we are to honor the core ideas central to defining patient experience as *the sum of all interactions, shaped by an organization's culture, that influence patient perceptions across* the *continuum of care*, we must also acknowledge its evolution. If we are to truly understand its impact, we must recognize all it now encompasses. If we are to elevate our humanity, then we must work to transform human experience in healthcare.

> *If we are to elevate our humanity, then we must work to transform human experience in healthcare.*

We invite healthcare professionals and experience champions globally to join us in that shared commitment to transforming human experience in healthcare. We hope you see this book as an inspirational, strategic, and practical guide— and are confident that we can bring the core ideas we share to life. In doing so, we will ensure that human experience is at the heart of healthcare for many years to come.

CHAPTER 1

An Integrated View of Experience

At its core, healthcare is about human beings caring for human beings. There is power in this statement—power that serves as a guiding force in the evolution of the healthcare-experience conversation. In this chapter, we frame experience as an expanding concept that first began with a singular, transactional view: that "healthcare" simply meant caring for patients. This narrow perspective of experience was not only limiting but also hindered our ability to provide true, measurable, and positive outcomes.

Applying the idea of human beings caring for human beings helps us broaden our approach to healthcare to one that is all-encompassing—one that is inclusive of patients, family members and care partners, the healthcare workforce, and the communities that healthcare organizations serve. With this perspective, it follows that a commitment to action on experience should be equally all-encompassing—one that extends from long before a patient selects an organization for care or treatment to well after they leave the clinical setting. It is also grounded in the idea that experience is not just a connected series of distinct transactions but rather a woven strand of relational encounters that people have with, and in, a healthcare organization across their personal healthcare journey. If we consider experience from this relational and holistic approach, we must both acknowledge and act on the idea that experience is not simply reflected in the results of a survey and instead is driven by an integrated effort that moves beyond just what organizations do to who they are.

This chapter frames the very idea of experience on which the remainder of the book is built. This framing will move us from the central idea of a core definition for experience to the guiding principles that help organizations gravitate from ideas to action. It will guide us from the integrated view reflected in an Experience Framework, including components that reflect and influence experience, to an expanded view of human experience. And it will ultimately be reflected in a community declaration for how we transform experience, along with a value case demonstrating the true return on human experience overall. But this journey, and by extension our story, begins with a definition.

DEFINING PATIENT EXPERIENCE

Though there is more consensus among healthcare organizations around the importance of experience, some continue to struggle to define what it truly means. Yet establishing a clear definition is essential for making meaningful progress in improving patient experience. Before The Beryl Institute had its first member, we realized that we needed to define "patient experience." We knew that in order to build a body of work around something, we had to first know what that something was. The definition we created with our community back in 2010 remains the foundation of all that we have done and continue to do.

The Beryl Institute defines "patient experience" as the sum of all interactions, shaped by an organization's culture, that influence patient perceptions across the continuum of care.[1] This definition, which will be further explored in Chapter 2, reflects a broad and encompassing nature of experience. It is grounded in all interactions driven by the people that comprise healthcare organizations and shaped by the cultures they build. Yet it must also be acknowledged that experience is primarily measured through the eyes of its recipient, be it the patient or long-term care resident, family members, loved ones, or friends in support. This means that every person has their own healthcare experience—clinically and non-clinically; through quality, safety, cost, and service-related touch points; and through the stories they hear from others. As such, in all that we do, it is *the patient's* perception of their experience that is essential.

As our work evolved, we discovered that we also needed methods to enact that definition. Our eight guiding principles emerged from this thought process and were then integrated into the creation of the Experience Framework that reflects the breadth of both what impacts and is impacted by experience. Our conversation then expanded to encompass human experience in healthcare and ultimately was formalized in the "Declaration for Human Experience." Each idea was combined with and built upon the one before it in a continuity of thought and work to provide the framing needed for the healthcare experience.

At the heart of how we turn these ideas to action are the guiding principles.

GUIDING PRINCIPLES

To address the question of what steps should be taken to move the definition of patient experience from words to action, we conducted a community-wide examination of organizational efforts. We did this with the intent of looking at the actions of successful organizations and the lessons learned from those still striving for excellence. The themes and common ideals that emerged led to a concise framework underlying patient experience success. This framework, which we termed the "Guiding Principles for Patient Experience Excellence," represents a set of actionable concepts central to achieving experience excellence.[2] These principles frame not only the healthcare experience but also this book in the chapters that follow.

We believe that organizations and systems committed to providing the best in experience will:

- develop a formal definition of experience that is understood and shared by all;
- identify and support accountable leadership with committed time and focused intent to shape, guide, and execute experience strategy;
- establish and reinforce a strong, vibrant, and positive organizational culture;
- understand and act on the needs and vulnerabilities of the healthcare workforce;
- implement a defined process for formal, intentional, and continuous partnerships with patients, families, and care partners;
- acknowledge that the healthcare experience reaches beyond clinical interactions to all touch points across the continuum of care;
- ensure an active commitment to health equity and access to care; and
- expand focus on health outcomes beyond treating illness to addressing the health and well-being of communities.[3]

Though not intended to be a list of specific tactics, these guiding principles represent a set of strategic considerations for action presented from two complementary perspectives. The first four principles represent concrete efforts that organizations can and should take to address their commitment to experience. These range from developing a formal definition and identifying specific leadership to building strong culture and establishing a clear process for patient and family input. The second four principles represent an opportunity to provide the strategic framing for experience excellence. These include a commitment to engaging all voices, recognizing the breadth of where experience happens, ensuring alignment and systemic focus, and moving to a model of community well-being.

Our intent in developing these guiding principles was to offer strategic actions and tangible points of focus that organizations can apply to drive experience efforts forward. In practice, as we saw how they conjoined and overlapped, merged and built upon each other, they guided us in creating an integrated Experience Framework.

EXPERIENCE FRAMEWORK

The experience journey we had been on as a community through the development of the guiding principles led us to a point where we could stand together in providing a formal frame to understand our opportunities and guide our actions. To reinforce the active and integrated nature of the concepts in our guiding principles and that are central to experience excellence, we took one more step and introduced the Experience Framework (Figure 1), again guided by the voices of our community. This framework was not designed simply as a call to action and a hope for a response but rather as a move to action in and of itself. We understood that when we align as a community around all that is fundamental to experience success and help others understand all that experience work encompasses, we could truly call ourselves a movement.

Using the Experience Framework provides strategic clarity and a means to identify where we are excelling (or where we have opportunities to address) and offers a structure through which knowledge, resources, and solutions can be aligned. This framing also helps in ensuring there is a comprehensive set of actions in place focused on the experience effort overall. Through this common framework, we found that we

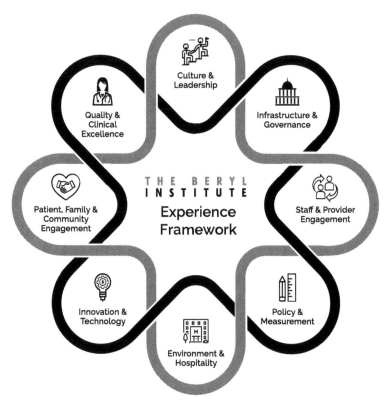

Figure 1. The Beryl Institute Experience Framework.

could create more efficient connections of needs to knowledge, strategies to resources, and opportunities to solutions. We could also expand our collective global dialogue through a common structure for focus and action.

The Experience Framework is built on eight strategic lenses, all of which address the factors that impact and influence experience and are simultaneously impacted and influenced by it. Each of the lenses is also accompanied by a statement of "why" rather than a definition. Our intention was not to create a static model of commonly accepted definitions but rather to introduce eight active lenses and the considerations for why they require our focus in any experience effort. The eight lenses and their why statements follow:

1. **Culture and leadership:** the foundation of any successful experience effort is set on what an organization is, its purpose and values, and how it is led.
2. **Infrastructure and governance:** effective experience efforts require both the right structures and processes by which to operate and communicate and formal guidance in place to ensure sustained strategic focus.
3. **Patient, family, and community engagement:** central to any experience effort are the voices of, contributions from, and partnerships with those receiving care and the community served.
4. **Staff and provider engagement:** caring for those delivering and supporting the delivery of care and reaffirming a connection to meaning and purpose is fundamental to the successful realization of a positive experience.
5. **Environment and hospitality:** the space in which a healthcare experience is delivered and the practices implemented to ensure a positive, comfortable, and compassionate encounter must be part of every effort.
6. **Innovation and technology:** as a focus on experience expands, it requires new ways of thinking and doing and the technologies and tools to ensure efficiencies, expand capacities, and extend boundaries of care.
7. **Policy and measurement:** experience is driven and influenced by external factors and systemic and financial realities and requires accepted and understood metrics to effectively measure outcomes and drive action.
8. **Quality and clinical excellence:** experience encompasses all an individual encounters and the expectations they have for safe, quality, reliable, and effective care focused on positively impacting health and well-being.[4]

Throughout each of these considerations, we stress that all voices are critical and matter in the experience conversation. This framework recognizes that no two individual experiences can or will ever be the same. As such, this is not intended as a one-size-fits-all solution but rather as a strategic framework to enable that level of individualization to be even more effective. It reaches well beyond the clinical experience of patients to the full extent of human experience in healthcare. To that end, the framework represents a range of perspectives and honors the breadth of those perspectives in its considerations. It does so while intentionally helping to align and support the broader strategic and operational items that impact experience endeavors. It also guided us in evolving our own framing.

EVOLVING FROM PATIENT EXPERIENCE TO HUMAN EXPERIENCE

As others aligned themselves around a common understanding of experience, we too began to see from varying perspectives both all that influences it and, in turn, all that it influences. The reality that you cannot isolate the experience of those whom healthcare serves from those who show up to serve every day, along with the communities in which they serve, has become increasingly apparent.

The realization that the experience of the healthcare workforce is important is not new. Conversations on employee engagement, staff morale, and culture have long been part of organizational efforts. However, they have been seen as distinct from, rather than integrated with, the experience that healthcare organizations look to provide.

We also came to see how intricately linked healthcare organizations are to the communities in which they operate and whom they serve. The realities that impact the broader sense of community health and well-being are a context that impacts how experiences are delivered and perceived in healthcare organizations. They do not operate distinctly from, but rather in concert with, their communities. Communities are where both patients and the workforce come from and go back to. They are directly impacted by the care provided and influence how care is delivered. Communities are where the stories that people share about their healthcare experience are told and amplified.

The realization that the experience of the healthcare workforce is important is not new. Conversations on employee engagement, staff morale, and culture have long been part of organizational efforts. However, they have been seen as distinct from, rather than integrated with, the experience that healthcare organizations look to provide.

We found that we could no longer have experience conversations effectively without this awareness and understanding of the workforce and community impacts to, and influences on, experience. This recognition of the needs and influence of patients, the healthcare workforce, and the communities that healthcare organizations serve catalyzed a shift in our thinking—a conversation on experience had to be broader if we were going to be true to what experience was about and what it needed to encompass. As such, we shifted from the more limited approach to experience in the past to this more inclusive, holistic approach going forward. In line with our comprehensive approach, we expanded the language we use, transitioning from just using the term "patient experience" to talking about the broader "human experience" in healthcare.

Recognizing the vital roles of healthcare workers, family members, care partners, and communities, this broader perspective warmly embraces all stakeholders in the continuum of care. It also underlines the critical elements that organizations must now consider when creating a definition for themselves that is shared and understood by all. Human experience integrates the sum of all interactions and every encounter among patients, families and care partners, the healthcare workforce, and the communities in which healthcare organizations operate. It is driven by the culture of healthcare organizations and systems that work tirelessly to support an ecosystem that operates across and even beyond the edges of the care continuum into the communities they serve and the ever-changing environmental landscapes in which they are situated. Human experience in healthcare ultimately is built on the core of patient experience itself.

When we return to the core ideas of interactions that people have in healthcare, the culture of the healthcare organizations we build, the continuum of care across which healthcare operates, and the perceptions that patients, family members, and care partners have of their healthcare encounters, we have a framework on which to explore the healthcare experience. It reflects a set of concepts and core elements on which experience strategy and practice can be and has been built. It is in the application of these very ideas that the boundaries of experience itself have been pushed.

The definition first created in 2010 is grounded in two operational realities: (1) experience happens at each point of interaction (primarily between two people) and (2) experience is driven by the cultures we build in organizations. These ideas tied the definition to the guiding principles, the guiding principles to the Experience Framework, and ultimately to this expanded view of human experience, in which we address the patient, workforce, and community experience as inextricably linked. For us, the next logical step was to have the community make a commitment to acting on this framework of experience.

DECLARATION FOR HUMAN EXPERIENCE

Once we understood that the human experience model reflects the best state for experience, we knew we needed to elevate the commitment of organizations around the world. We saw healthcare facilities that were struggling with overcapacity, staffing shortages, and supply issues, leading to overwhelmed and exhausted healthcare workers. At the same time, systemic disparities and inequities continued to significantly impact access to care, affordability, and quality outcomes. We saw ourselves at a critical inflection point.

We knew it was time to put a stake in the ground around three core commitments that were grounded on a fourth, one that reflects the foundational value of The Beryl Institute itself: collaboration and shared learning. In the "Declaration for Human Experience," we set forth a call to action for the global healthcare community to commit to the following:

- Acknowledge and dismantle systemic racism and prejudice, tackle disparities, and provide the highest-quality, most equitable care possible.
- Understand and act on the needs and vulnerabilities of the healthcare workforce to honor their commitment and reaffirm and reenergize their purpose.
- Recognize and maintain a focus on what matters most to patients, their family members, and care partners to ensure unparalleled care and a commitment to health and well-being.
- Collaborate through shared learning within and between organizations, systems, and the broader healthcare continuum to forge a bold new path to a more human-centered, equitable, and effective healthcare system.[5]

In many ways, this declaration takes us back to the very roots of The Beryl Institute community. Reaffirming that the fourth commitment to learning and collaboration has been our foundational value from the start, it is important to note that it was our hope to create a space where this could happen that sparked the birth of the Institute community. As such, coming together in this commitment via the "Declaration for Human Experience" felt as if we were coming full circle—and in a way, we had. We are not suggesting that the evolving work of healthcare experience will ever have a conclusion, but our work, our framing, and our community had reached a new level of understanding and collaboration. This collective effort signified a milestone where our shared goals and values and a unified vision converged to drive meaningful change through a commitment to a specific call to action, as human beings caring for human beings, around the world.

THE VALUE CASE FOR THE RETURN ON EXPERIENCE

The essential premise of this book is that if we commit to human experience, we will see true value in the outcomes for healthcare organizations. Traditionally, that value was harder to define, as experience was viewed more narrowly—from patient registration to discharge, attempting to fit within the specific departmental silos where each segment focused on its own goals or as simply the results of satisfaction surveys. Though this approach may have been logistically sound, it did not align with how patients actually experience healthcare.

The concept of value in healthcare also tends to focus primarily on healthcare outcomes per dollar spent. However, the reality is that healthcare is a complex system driven by far more than how much is spent or even the very patient outcomes we strive to achieve. It is driven by how healthcare organizations engage with patients as people, care for their workforce, and address the needs of the communities they serve. To that end, value is not solely about dollars or clinical outcomes but also about the comprehensive healthcare experience through which a much broader set of outcomes is achieved.

Examining the impacts of human experience as an integrated effort, we can see how it positively contributes to a wide range of desired outcomes. This broad focus on human experience has us consider the patient, care partner, workforce, and community experiences not individually but in connection with one another. An investment in experience has a positive, measurable impact on the overall objectives of healthcare organizations, driving value in four key areas:[6]

Workforce/Team Value

- **Vibrant culture.** Building and sustaining a positive experience environment contributes to a vibrant culture—one in which organizations benefit from increased attraction and retention of team members and increased team engagement and loyalty, all of which support stronger, more sustainable outcomes.
- **Team well-being.** A healthy workforce in mind, body, and spirit is more important now than ever. A focus on team well-being reinforces purpose, instills joy, promotes safety, and secures commitment to, and trust in, an organization.

Patient, Family, and Care Partner Value

- **Clinical outcomes.** A commitment to experience acknowledges that safe care is an integral part of that experience. Managing processes effectively, communicating openly, and listening to each patient's perspective of safety are all outcomes of an experience effort.
- **Positive engagement.** Engaging patients and care partners as co-designers of their care experience is essential to any experience effort. Ensuring a clear

willingness to listen, while communicating in ways people can understand, means ensuring greater engagement and increased value.

Organizational/Business Value

- **Brand strength.** Strong experience efforts frame the stories people will tell, drive loyalty to an organization, and encourage patient choice. Collectively, these significantly increase brand strength and community reputation.
- **Operational efficiency.** Operational efficiency is about more than cutting expenses. It is delivered through people who are clear on their expectations and grounded in open and honest communication processes, providing the foundation for financial viability.

Community/Consumer Value

- **Access and community wellness.** The impact that healthcare organizations have in their communities is a key value realized in experience. A commitment to experience calls for active efforts to ensure expanded access to care and a commitment to elevating the health of the communities in which they operate.
- **Ensured equity.** An effective experience strategy can only be fully effective if it works for all in the community a healthcare organization serves. In this way, it helps ensure equity, creates easier, more accessible paths to care and treatment, and works to dismantle the disparities still evident in the day-to-day workings of healthcare.

An integrated experience strategy not only has a broad impact on value in these ways but also aligns the actions and efforts of an organization. For example, though effective communication may be a tool taught specifically for team building and workforce well-being, it is also a resource that supports how people communicate better with patients and care partners, with a direct impact on reducing mistakes and positively affecting quality outcomes. It is critical that improvement efforts and experience strategies are recognized as more than addressing one specific need by looking at the broader impact they can have on the overall value an organization provides.

A focus on experience helps us achieve everything we strive for in healthcare. It enhances outcomes for patients, cultivates a positive work environment, builds trust within communities, and ensures financial viability and operational sustainability. It also drives quality, safety, and workforce engagement while boosting reputation and consumer loyalty. Healthcare organizations now have a tremendous opportunity to evolve, just as our own experience journey has. By focusing on the overall human experience and breaking down silos, you can enhance both the quality of care and operational efficiency. This approach not only benefits patients but also strengthens an organization's business model, ensuring sustainability and success in the ever-evolving healthcare landscape. Committing to experience in this way, where you include patient, workforce, and community engagement, means transcending short-term objectives to authentically address and reach an organization's long-term vision.

What you will find in the chapters that follow is a guide to moving your organization forward in realizing this value for your patients, your workforce, and your community. Though each of us may chart slightly different paths, choose different tactics, or even prioritize different strategies, this guide will provide a general direction for where the industry can, and must, go in its commitment to transform human experience in healthcare. Aside from the fact that improving experience significantly improves all these outcomes, it is simply the right thing to do. And similar to our beginnings at The Beryl Institute, we must first start with a definition.

CHAPTER 2

Defining Experience Is Step One

> ## Guiding Principle: Develop a formal definition of experience that is understood and shared by all
>
> **Key Takeaways**
> 1. A clear and shared definition of experience serves as a "true north" in guiding all organizational efforts.
> 2. A definition must reflect the comprehensive and integrated nature of the healthcare experience to inform and guide strategy.
> 3. A definition must be more than words; it should be an active and strategic way to engage people in working toward a common purpose.

If we believe that experience—the integrated delivery of quality, safety, and service in care—is, at its core, the very strategic footing on which we build healthcare organizations and our capacity to deliver the best in outcomes, then we must clearly define what that experience will be for our organization. In doing so, we leave much less to chance, we clarify expectations for all engaged, and we align our actions with focus and direction. This is the essence of this first guiding principle. If we are to address experience in any healthcare organization, it's important that we:

- are clear about what we mean;
- ensure that people understand what we mean; and
- align, incent, and ensure that action is taken to fulfill what we mean in all that we do.

However, without first having a definition, we cannot do any of this; we would have no basis for action without understanding what that action is intended to accomplish. In this respect, we also offer a word of caution. Simply defining "experience" without taking any action to back it up is merely putting words on paper. If there is no commitment to action, a definition in its own right is merely decoration. But when those words are combined with actions that are intended to advance those sentiments, and are reinforced in the commitments, statements, and efforts of leaders, the potential to move an organization forward is limitless.

In practice, the concept of patient experience is often discussed with little more explanation than what the term itself represents. This is despite the fact that the term's use continues to grow in the general healthcare vernacular as well as in the realm of both clinical practice and research. In the United States, this increase has largely been exemplified in shifts in public policy and associated measures that have had an impact on incentives and reimbursements. It has also been the result of the corresponding expansion of the consumer mindset in healthcare. Through our research, we have further found, especially from a global perspective, an awakening due to these factors that is reflected in organizations and their leaders acknowledging that ensuring a positive patient experience is just the right thing to do. Most of the world's attention on this issue is grounded in this idea. With this as a backdrop, we can say with confidence that experience is now a top priority for healthcare leaders.

Organizations are now acting with more intention from the perspective that, in order to provide a good experience, they need to first know what that is, to be able to express it with clarity, and to have it be understood by others. We have consistently asked our community the question, "Does your organization have a formal definition of experience?" every two years since 2011. Initially, only 27 percent reported having one. That was followed by a jump to 45 percent in just two years and then a steady ebb and flow through the years that followed. As of 2023, that initial percentage had nearly doubled to 56 percent.[7] And though we are encouraged to see this type of increase in 12 years, 44 percent of organizations have not yet defined what patient experience means to them.[8] An opportunity still clearly remains. And to reaffirm, without a definition, how do you ultimately know where you are going?

The irony is that while everyone is in a rush to develop a plan to provide a positive experience, few can express what that actually means for their own organization. As such, efforts often fall short due to this lack of clarity and alignment. This isn't surprising. How can you frame an effective strategy around something without first defining it and being clear on the shared idea and purpose?

This challenge is one we too experienced in the very early days of The Beryl Institute. We knew that if we were to be a community focused on experience, we needed to first define that experience. We needed to be clear on what we meant and ensure it was shared and understood—and that it provided clarity and direction of our community as we built our resources and committed ourselves to growth. That realization led to conversations with some of the initial participants in our community and to what is now the Institute's definition, which we introduced in Chapter 1: "Patient experience is the sum of all interactions, shaped by an organization's culture, that influence patient perceptions across the continuum of care."[9]

Having this definition in place allowed us to develop framing and a methodology around it. We did this primarily through our guiding principles, the Experience Framework, and the "Declaration for Human Experience," which cumulatively have provided the foundation for all the work we have done since. However, we would not have had the ability to do any of this without first having a clear and shared definition of "patient experience."

ESTABLISH A FORMAL DEFINITION

We believe that the core ideas found in our community definition—interactions, culture, perceptions, and a view across the continuum of care—are indispensable in defining patient experience. This belief has been further cemented through the vast use of the definition throughout our global community. Over a decade after we first set forth the definition of patient experience, we continue to see an incredible rate of adoption and adaptation. It now appears in applications around the world, in multiple languages. And though many adopt it wholly without changing a word, others have adapted it to apply these concepts in a way that best supports their own strategies and objectives. For example, the largest health system in the world, the Veterans Health Administration (VHA), part of the U.S. Department of Veterans Affairs, defines patient experience as "the sum of all interactions shaped by the organization's culture that influence veterans' and their families' perceptions along their health care journey."[10] In this adaptation, they customized their definition based specifically on whom they serve, while the core elements of the totality of all interactions, shaped by the culture and across the entire journey, remain the same.

As we see adaptations of the definition like the one above applied, from some of the world's largest healthcare systems to some of the smaller local healthcare provider organizations, it's clear that it is not the exactness of the definition that has moved people but rather its simplicity and the recognition of the shared concepts that align experience efforts. Our hope in defining experience was, and still is, that this definition would create a shared understanding and common framework to be used as others take action in their own organizations. We also wanted it to serve as the standard for how we support and advocate for the creation of a positive experience across all healthcare organizations. Our intent has always been not to land on a static definition but to create a dynamic and living framework that would evolve to honor the active nature that experience represents.

Though we invite you to adapt or adopt our definition, like so many others have, what's most important is that you establish a formal definition for your organization and that it is understood and shared by all. The core elements should be something your organization can not only get behind but also commit to and own going forward.

REEXAMINING THE CORE ELEMENTS

In suggesting that you consider adapting or adopting our community definition, we understand the importance of examining the core elements that comprise it. Oftentimes, we need to look back in order to look forward with clarity and intention. A few years after the introduction of the definition, members of our community dug deeper into the concepts that can and should frame a formal definition in a landmark article in the *Patient Experience Journal*. The extensive review and synthesis of literature spanning 14-plus years focused on recurrent instances of terminology and constructs that could be generalized into the core elements of what comprise a comprehensive definition of patient experience.[11]

This work revealed foundational concepts at the core of the evolving conversation of experience and have continued to hold true. The core concepts assert, and we reinforce again here, that experience:

- as an idea crosses the continuum of care and is not just limited to a specific care setting or just the clinical encounter of care but to all touch points through which one encounters a healthcare organization;
- is not simply about quantitative measures or survey results that may capture insights into specific points or parts of a care journey but must be understood for all the interactions one has with a healthcare organization and the impact those have on an individual, their family, and/or care partners;
- remains grounded in the expectations and perceptions of those engaging with healthcare organizations; people in healthcare organizations come with a certain set of beliefs or hopes, and through their experiences and observations, frame realities that make each and every encounter unique;
- is built on the principles of patient-centered care and patient and family partnership and engagement; the essential approaches reflected in these concepts must reach beyond just the clinical setting itself;
- is individual and personalized, and the actions taken and processes put in place must support the uniqueness of each person's encounter in the face of seeking process generalization and efficiencies; and
- is much more than satisfaction, as satisfaction is an indicator of moments in time, but experience captures all someone encounters, the perceptions they take with them, and the stories they tell as a result.[12]

In reflecting on this initial framing and the conversation on experience, we firmly believe that these core concepts continue to hold true today. They shape the identification and reinforcement of the key elements we believe essential to the definition of experience presented more than a decade ago and seen abundantly actualized in practice since. The core elements and supporting concepts represent a simple but broad lens through which one can define experience.

The sum of all interactions, organizational culture, and patient (including family and care partner) perceptions across the continuum of care, supported by the foundational themes of integration, person-centeredness, and patient and family partnership, all remain essential to what experience is today. They remain purposefully simple and clear, broad, inclusive, open, and challenging, as these ideas do not represent a basic checklist for how to "do" experience (as many seek). Rather, experience is reflected in how an organization lives and breathes and in how it engages those it cares for, well before any clinical interaction and well after. It is why we believe these concepts remain essential, while recognizing that the notion of experience itself has appropriately evolved.

IMPACTS OF HAVING A DEFINITION

When you create a shared definition of experience in your organization, you set yourself up for success. With a common language based on the terms you use, your people can understand it, share it, and make strategic choices based on it. They can better understand what you intend, so they know where you're going collectively as an organization and how they can each individually contribute to success.

We believe that the process of aligning people around the definition can, in many ways, be as important as the words themselves. Organizations can look to the framing of their own definition as a unique opportunity to clarify what is central to the type of healthcare experience they hope to deliver and/or would wish to receive. It is a chance for organizational alignment and understanding, as well as an opportunity for clarity and shared ownership.

> *Organizations can look to the framing of their own definition as a unique opportunity to clarify what is central to the type of healthcare experience they hope to deliver and/or would wish to receive.*

In the business of healthcare, there is no more central purpose than the care and well-being of those we serve. We ultimately strive to provide the best in quality, safety, and service—the very outcomes that drive healthcare providers and support staff; inspire leaders; relieve families, care partners, and friends; and heal and support patients. These concepts in total are the experience that patients and families hope for, anticipate, and remember long after their clinical encounter is over. They also help frame the stories people tell others about their encounters with our healthcare organizations every day. They are the foundations of experience, and in order to be effective, this purpose must be clear to all, which can only be achieved through a definition of what that is.

It is here, as well, where we see the importance of reinforcing the foundational concepts in the definition as relevant beyond just the concept of the "patient experience" to the broader concept of the "human experience," to which we have committed as an organization. At the core of the definition has always been the idea of culture—how we create strong organizations that care for those who work in healthcare—and the reality that experience reaches across the continuum of care into the communities that healthcare organizations serve. The very idea of experience links the patient, workforce, and community experience. The definitions we create must also consider this important integration if we are to achieve the best in experience excellence overall.

In considering the impact and purpose of definition, we reinforce that ensuring clarity of both direction and purpose that is understood and shared by all in it is fundamental to building, leading, and sustaining a successful organization. This holds true not only for overall organizational strategy but also for the critical work an organization takes on in reaching for its vision and realizing its objectives. To do this effectively, you first must understand what it is you are looking to achieve and where it is you are striving to go in your own organization. In the context of experience, you can only do that by defining specifically what the experience is you are seeking to provide in every moment, every day.

CREATING A DEFINITION

As we discussed in the beginning of this chapter, words without action are merely decorative. You need to take action, including the very initial act of creating a definition for your organization based on what patient experience means to you. This includes taking the following steps:

1. Commit to developing a definition for your own organization.
2. Consider how you may want to adapt or adopt the existing definition developed by The Beryl Institute community.
3. Engage patient and family voices around what is important to them in an experience with your organization.
4. Engage team voices in why providing an experience is important to them and what it means to be able to deliver on the experience defined.

5. Analyze the feedback received and work to simplify these concepts or tie them into why the definition you adapt or adopt enables you to achieve those things.
6. Determine the core elements that should be included in your definition—whether they are based on The Beryl Institute's core elements or some variation thereof.
7. Draft a clear and concise definition that captures the essence of what patient experience means at your organization.
8. Share the draft of the definition to ensure there is clarity around your intent, get feedback, and revise, as needed.
9. Finalize your organization's definition of experience.
10. Share the definition internally and externally and embed it into the organization's culture by incorporating it into policies, procedures, and performance metrics.

These recommended actions are intended to provide you with stepping stones in your quest to create a definition of experience for your organization—one that you can stand proudly upon and build from.

From the start, we have believed that there is no single model for how to address experience. In much the same way, there is not necessarily only one definition. You certainly do not need to use the community definition; however, we believe strongly that the concepts that comprise it are essential to shaping experience success.

This was the central idea we used in crafting the original definition with broad but essential concepts back in 2010. And we have, since those very early days, been clear in calling for organizations to adapt or adopt these ideas or create a definition of their own. This is the first of our guiding principles for an important reason: If you are not clear on what you are trying to achieve, on where you are wanting to go, how will you ever get there? How will you ever encourage your people and your organization to go with you?

Healthcare organizations, just like each of us, need a true north. Having one ensures clarity around what we seek to achieve and helps us build shared paths to get there. It provides a space where leadership and the workforce can align in action. The absence of this clarity leaves organizations at risk before they ever start. Tactics applied without a clear purpose or direction can lead us in multiple directions. Rather than tightening the intention and focus of an organization, it can literally pull at and unravel its seams.

The bottom line is that having a definition matters, and ensuring that it is shared and understood by all is a must if you are truly seeking experience success. It is the foundation on which everything we share follows—the cornerstone on which you build an experience for patients and care partners, your workforce, and the communities you serve.

What Is the Impact?

- Stronger alignment around common purpose
- Increased connection between purpose and action
- Expanded understanding of what experience encompasses

CHAPTER 3

Accountable Leadership Is Essential

Guiding Principle: Identify and support accountable leadership with committed time and focused intent to shape, guide, and execute experience strategy

Key Takeaways

1. Experience leaders must have operational accountability and influence and reside in, or have direct access to, the C-suite to ensure alignment and integration with all organizational efforts.
2. Experience leaders must be directly engaged in an organization's strategic planning process to ensure that experience is a primary driver of desired outcomes.
3. Though experience leadership is a must, the presence of an individual leader does not relieve members of an organization from the responsibility of delivering a positive experience.

Underlying experience excellence is the consistent need to identify and support accountable leadership. With committed time and focused intent, those in leadership positions have the ability to shape, guide, and execute experience strategy. Focused leadership is a statement of commitment to the importance of experience efforts. Just as there are other strategically defined roles committed to driving outcomes, such as vice presidents of human resources and chief financial officers, it follows that organizations should also choose to identify an individual or individuals with strategic accountability for experience.

This role is increasingly being filled by chief experience officers (CXOs), typically reporting to the C-suite, but there are many other ways accountable leadership can be structured just as effectively. We would never suggest that there is just one model that every organization should follow. Such a proposition is counter to the core values of an experience effort that emphasizes meeting people, including your teams, where they are, understanding the context in which they operate, applying what truly matters most to them, and using the feedback received to design and improve efforts.

Just as there are other strategically defined roles committed to driving outcomes, such as vice presidents of human resources and chief financial officers, it follows that organizations should also choose to identify an individual or individuals with strategic accountability for experience.

We would also be remiss if we failed to acknowledge the challenges that healthcare faces globally, particularly in terms of resource constraints, financial challenges, workforce depletion, and burnout. However, these challenges render decisions on experience strategy and how to structure an experience effort even more significant. For example, there is a true cost-benefit conversation to be had on why a commitment to experience matters and why an investment in structure is important.

In responsibly managing resources, it is better to act with intent toward desired outcomes—clinical quality, financial viability, workforce engagement, equity, loyalty, and reputation—versus leaving those outcomes to chance. A commitment to experience is not a strategic afterthought or a plan for how to make an experience effort fit into strategy. Rather, it is intentionally focused on the idea that experience is the primary driver of the outcomes that organizations seek to achieve. As such, experience considerations must be part of all strategic planning.

Consider examples such as Ritz Carlton's commitment to its guests, Zappos's support of its customers, the encounters that families have with Disney, or the unique nature of shopping at Trader Joe's. The explicit commonality of these organizations is the tangible and clear appeal of the experience they provide and the underlying commitment they make to the people who work for them.

What you do not see, and what these organizations do not take for granted, is the infrastructure of commitment and investment it takes to strategically and consistently deliver on the experience they vow to provide. From training and resources to reinforcement and rewards, these organizations and others committed to experience excellence put the pieces in place to ensure consistency in their efforts to achieve the results they seek. There is no reason to do any less in healthcare.

A GLOBAL INQUIRY INTO EFFECTIVE LEADERSHIP STRUCTURE

There has been an emerging and active conversation among members of The Beryl Institute's global community about how others are structuring their experience efforts. In the paper "The Human Experience Imperative: Practical insights for executives on organizational strategy, structure and impact," members of the Institute community explored the types of experience structures that organizations are putting in place and the implications and impact of this commitment.[13] This inquiry was inspired and supported by members of the Institute's Experience Leaders Circle (XLC), a group representing organizations with designated senior-level experience leaders.

Forty-two organizations provided input covering leadership roles, department range, intra-organization collaboration, engagement of patient and family advisors, and more.[14] The organizations that contributed reflected the range of current healthcare organizations from integrated and multinational delivery systems to single hospital organizations to managed-care organizations. They included organizations across multiple continents, ranging in size from 1,500 to more than 50,000 employees. It should also be noted that many of the organizations included in the inquiry are already organizations with a commitment to having an experience leader. This allowed for insights into how organizations making that commitment are approaching this work while still revealing a range of differences and considerations to explore.

AN INVESTMENT IN EXPERIENCE LEADERSHIP AND STRUCTURE IS NEEDED

Our ongoing research shows that organizations are investing in experience leadership overall. In the "State of Human Experience 2023" study, 63 percent of respondents reported having some level of experience leader in place.[15] Though this appears promising on the surface, the commitment, which is often limited to a single leader who is given the full burden of experience outcomes, itself is not enough.

In organizations with only a single experience leader, the scope of what can be addressed is significantly limited, often leading to an experience strategy that is only focused on a singular goal. This is not to suggest that this model is wrong. For many organizations, this may be driven by their size, strategic choices, and/or budget constraints. However, it is important to understand that organizations whose experience structure is limited must still find ways to effectively lead an integrated experience effort. A single person tasked with moving a single metric (or metrics) misses the larger strategic opportunities realized in a comprehensive experience strategy.

Julie Oehlert, CXO, ECU Health, sums it up: "The world and all the potential patients within it are begging for healthcare systems that are wired to deliver safe, quality care with love and human care. Achieving this requires rethinking, retooling, and restructuring how hospitals, health systems, and other health entities' structure, support, and lead experience offices and teams. Experience professionals can fill the roles and lead a variety of functions and services that benefit from knowledge in hospitality, caring science, and service recovery."[16]

Experience leadership is a must, and whether it's a single leader or one with a more extensive team, that presence does not relieve others who work in a healthcare organization from the responsibility of delivering a positive experience. Though experience strategy should be framed and guided by defined leadership, it must be owned and executed by all. This is the premise in the statement "the sum of all interactions" from the definition of patient experience. Every touch point and every encounter one has with a healthcare organization matters. Therefore, every member of an organization, from those at the point of care to those supporting behind the scenes to the senior-most leader, all must feel and act with a sense of ownership for the experience their organization provides.

Building further on the statement "the sum of all interactions," an investment in experience needs to strategically focus on what it will take to ensure positive interactions. As interactions are driven by an organization's culture, the investment it takes to attract, develop, retain, and maintain good talent and making the commitment to ensure a strong, positive culture are not disparate from an experience strategy. For this reason, experience structures need to be integrated in how an organization operates and how experience leaders must be fully engaged in strategy development. Their efforts not only impact how care partners interact with patients but also help set the cultural framework supporting a strong and positive culture of experience for both those receiving and those delivering care. It is therefore important that these experience leaders have access to or a presence in the C-suite.

EXPERIENCE LEADERS SHOULD RESIDE IN THE C-SUITE (OR HAVE DIRECT ACCESS TO IT)

The individual who leads experience for an organization is not a figurehead but rather an active leader who both ensures that the voice of the patient is present in all organizational decisions and reinforces the importance of an integrated strategy that elevates human experience. C-suite presence is essential to make sure there is alignment with other strategic efforts, such as quality and safety, marketing and digital engagement, environmental decisions, training, or employee engagement. Experience is a throughline that must be connected to the full range of strategic discussions a healthcare organization undertakes.

Though all organizations in the "Human Experience Imperative" study had a senior experience leader, there was some variation in their titles, from CXO to chief patient experience officer to SVP or VP of patient experience.[17] Many organizations are also still considering how to elevate the experience leader role they currently have, as many still have positions at the director or manager level. Ultimately, how the role is structured and where it resides in an organization has significant implications on the impact it can have.

In determining where senior experience leaders reside, we still found some variation. Most in our study now report directly to the chief executive officer (CEO) or someone reporting to the CEO (again, noting that this study was specifically of those organizations with senior experience leaders). Still others report to safety/quality leaders, human resources, or the chief nursing officer (CNO). About half remarked that, as senior experience leaders, they participate in regular executive/C-suite leadership meetings in which experience strategy is discussed and developed.[18]

Though not every organization will make the experience leader a C-suite role, we reinforce our belief that if experience is a key strategy for organizations, the experience leaders must either reside in or have direct access to the C-suite, as they play a key role in creating, integrating, and sustaining an organization's strategy. As such, they must be in a position to most effectively do so.

EXPERIENCE LEADERS SHOULD DRIVE THE DEVELOPMENT AND EXECUTION OF STRATEGY AND CULTURE

Building on the suggested placement of the experience leader at a senior organizational level, it is critical that they are engaged directly in both strategy and culture development. Returning to the definition of patient experience, the experience provided in any organization is "shaped by the culture" it builds and sustains. Though all organizations have a culture, some still leave culture to chance by lacking intentional planning. Effective experience strategies must be built on a planned and well-established culture built on clear expectations and a shared commitment.

This intentional choice calls for executive collaboration and strategic intent as well as an elevation of the experience conversation to the executive level. This is not just about an organization saying that it has such a role or even what that role's placement in an organization is, especially just to check a box; rather, it is about the intention of and accountability placed in the role to contribute to and help frame strategy and culture.

In committing to a strategic view of experience, this must reach beyond the executive team to organization governance as well. As finance, quality, and human resources may have board-level committees, the conversation on experience and culture must be elevated to that same level. The senior experience leader should be the champion in this governance structure.

A powerful example of this idea at work was shared by Shannon Connor Phillips. During her tenure as chief quality and experience officer at Intermountain Health, she helped guide an organizational shift in focus to one on experience as foundational. "We started with the premise that everybody has a quality department, but let's turn that upside down and start with experience," she reveals. "Of course, we attended to quality and doing no harm, and we started with caring and human connection." This shift was amplified by executive leadership and permeated throughout the organization and has led to great success within the organization. Phillips noted that when other organizations saw increases in harm during the height of the COVID-19 pandemic, Intermountain Health actually saw decreases.

In healthcare organizations, stated priorities garner attention, needed resources, and larger strategic commitments, so elevating experience to the highest strategic levels is critical; the senior experience leader is key to driving this. Elevating experience also presents a critical opportunity to address the next consideration: how to measure experience success.

EXPERIENCE LEADERS MUST ADDRESS MORE THAN JUST SURVEY METRICS

The measures of experience matter. Yet, all too often, the metrics collected from patient experience surveys are the only data considered. This is a far too narrow view that leaves organizations at great risk of missing all that influences the experience they provide. Patient survey data, such as the Centers for Medicare & Medicaid Services' Hospital Consumer Assessment of Healthcare Providers and Systems (HCAHPS) survey results for hospitals in the United States, does not equal experience; it reflects only one part of it.

Organizations should refrain, wherever possible, from equating experience solely with the collection and reporting of these metrics or other rankings or ratings. Improving survey scores is not an experience strategy. It is simply an indicator that an experience strategy may have some impact.

Relegating the role of experience in an organization to a single leader or experience office solely responsible for capturing and reporting scores misinforms the organization on the true extent of experience. It minimizes the sum of all interactions to snapshots of distinct and potentially disparate moments and events. At the same time, experience leaders and teams have a significant opportunity to champion innovative collection methods to capture and act on the voice of the patient. Opportunities for further digitization and personalization of experience, point of care, real-time feedback, and other efforts are expanding as organizations seek the best ways to measure experience success.

Great efforts are underway to find more functional, practical, actionable, and comparable means to gauge (and share) experience success and identify where positive impacts are being made. Data sharing occurs through multiple means. Distribution of data via reports is complemented by more interactive processes, such as reporting at unit- or department-level meetings and at larger facility-level town halls, including capturing and sharing patient and family stories and other means to reflect the realities of people's experience overall. Understanding that experience is about more than just metrics is fundamental to broader strategic success.

At the same time, without these measures, organizations would be hard pressed to capture the real impact a commitment to experience can have. Though the survey metrics are one means to do so, ensuring that experience leaders and offices have broader operational accountability also provides an opportunity to show impact.

EXPERIENCE LEADERS MUST HAVE OPERATIONAL ACCOUNTABILITY AND REACH

This idea is at the heart of how organizations are structuring successful experience efforts. It builds on the key strategic considerations previously mentioned to reinforce the essential elements needed for experience success. First, an experience office needs a defined team and budget. About two-thirds of those replying to the XLC structure inquiry noted the name of the function as being a variation of "Office of Patient Experience," "Patient Experience Department," or just "Patient Experience," while a few have an organizational branded experience department, such as "Veterans Experience Office" or "The Sharp Experience."[19]

We have seen experience efforts structured in a number of ways as well, with some centralized at a system level while others have distributed models with roles dispersed across an organization. Some also have hybrid models with both centralized (corporate resources) and local champions. Specifically in our study, experience offices ranged in size in terms of people directly reporting to the senior experience leader, yet most offices had six or more people identified as directly responsible for patient experience who report to a senior experience leader. Though it may not be possible in all larger structures, it is suggested that experience-related roles report in some capacity, either directly or indirectly, to a senior experience leader, as the disconnect of roles can impact consistency, strategic alignment, communication, and key outcomes including clinical quality, financial viability, equity, loyalty, and reputation—not to mention the bottom line.

Additionally, we suggest that experience structures include any operational functions that can impact experience outcomes. Ensuring operational accountability guarantees that an experience leader has regular influence on—and input from—operations. The scope and scale of what is included in experience functions is expanding as well. While we see experience structures include traditionally related experience functions, with direct accountability over measurement, patient and family advisor engagement, and service excellence, we also see experience functions expanding.[20]

Components of experience structure now typically include extended services such as concierge services, volunteer services, patient advocacy, and language services.[21] They are also now including areas such as patient education, arts in medicine, call-center services, community relations, spiritual care, and training and development.[22]

This expanding diversity in what experience efforts now include reinforces the central point that there is not a one-size-fits-all model. Experience efforts are broad yet also integrated with a singular goal to ensure the best in human experience for both all who are cared for by and all who work in a healthcare organization. Consider an approach that fits your organization, your culture, and your people that will enable you to realize the outcomes you seek to achieve.

EXPERIENCE LEADERS SERVE THE ROLE OF CHAMPION FOR HUMAN EXPERIENCE AND BOUNDARY SPANNER

An experience mission links patient voice to actions to outcome; it elevates cultural strategy as an experience influencer, ensures that governance is aware and invested, and commits to a broader focus on human experience, elevating issues of equity and inclusion and the broader community impact that healthcare organizations can have. Experience leaders and the offices they lead are champions for human experience. No experience effort can be fully successful without this integrated focus. In fact, in our inquiry of XLC members, fewer than half said that their department is focused on patient experience efforts only, while around a third reported having accountability for both patient and workforce experience. This reflects that there is still work to do in expanding the integration of experience as a comprehensive strategy.

We see experience leaders as boundary spanners in their organization, helping to weave disparate functions together for both those who seek and those who provide care, ensuring that experience leaders hold an organization-wide view versus that of only a specific function. This brings the critical considerations full circle, for if the experience leader is the primary integrator of essential functions driving human experience, their existence is a must.

Leaders must show a consistent commitment to engage and partner with the critical functions in their organizations. They must also champion the connection of these distinct segments under a broader commitment to the experience they provide. From diversity, equity, and inclusion (DEI) efforts to nursing and operations, marketing and communications to quality and human resources to learning and development, the role of the experience leader and their office is seen and positioned as the ultimate integrator of distinct functions under the broad and evolving concept of experience.

As we have previously shared, experience encompasses all the touch points one has on a healthcare journey, from before and after any specific clinical encounter and across all settings on the continuum of care. The recognition that an experience effort weaves these endeavors together is a fundamental idea that cannot be overlooked, especially when it comes to leadership, structure, and strategy. It is why a strategic focus on experience isn't just a nice to-do but rather is truly the best thing to do in terms of investing in a healthcare organization's purpose and future.

Jennifer Carron, CXO, BJC Health, may say it best: "The patient experience is a fundamental anchor in the longevity of an organization. Now is the time to lean into your patient experience leaders and team and focus on codesigning the experience so all who practice, work, and receive care are aligned. This cannot be executed by a single individual alone but rather by an entire team with the right resources and technology to bring your brand to life. Only then will you realize the outcomes you seek."[23]

STEPS TO TAKE IF CURRENTLY OPERATING WITHOUT AN EXPERIENCE FOCUS

You may be reading this thinking that the integrated structure we suggest is an idealistic model. While more and more organizations are reporting senior leader support, dedicated teams, and other resources at their disposal, that may not mirror your circumstance, so how does this apply to you? Where can you get started? What steps can you take to help your organization and leadership see a value in the investment in an experience effort? In many ways, answering those questions is the purpose of this book.

First, as you look to commit to an experience strategy and build an effective structure, ask yourself and your leaders what experience outcomes you hope to achieve. Broaden the perspective beyond simply survey metrics. In clarifying the broader opportunities of an experience commitment, you will begin to draw a path forward, framed on a series of foundational needs:

- The need to have dedicated leadership focused on experience excellence rather than leaving outcomes to chance.
- The need to intentionally integrate disparate efforts that impact the experience that people have in your organization and the need to establish the structure to make sure that happens.
- The need for someone to not only help champion the voice of patients but also listen to the needs of the workforce and engage the voice of your community to understand what is needed—and possible—for your organization to drive tangible and lasting improvement.

Establishing an integrated and committed leadership structure reinforces and ensures the value that a focus on experience brings to an organization. It is an investment that reaps great returns.

You can shape the experience journey in whatever way your organization needs, and you can start it at any time. The tangible impacts you will achieve with a commitment to experience excellence reinforce that though an investment in people and resources may be required, the return is exponentially greater. The central priority in healthcare remains providing the safest and highest-quality care possible—and a commitment to invest in experience, beginning with leadership, ensures just that.

What Is the Impact?

- Elevated strategic commitment to experience
- Integrated approach across an organization
- Expanded accountability for experience goals

CHAPTER 4

Culture Is the Foundation for Action

Guiding Principle: Establish and reinforce a strong, vibrant, and positive organizational culture

Key Takeaways

1. A strong, positive culture is the result of intentional choice and is cultivated through deliberate action and consistent reinforcement.
2. The commitment of leadership to model expected behaviors and actions is essential to establishing and sustaining a positive organizational culture.
3. A strong organizational culture both serves as the foundation from which people make choices and shapes their interactions with others.

Culture is the very foundation of human experience. It binds human values to crucial organizational components while simultaneously supporting the weight of all that must stand upon it. It is our belief that though there is no singular focus in achieving a positive human experience, if one had to be chosen, it would undeniably be culture. But this is not merely our contention. When asking exemplary healthcare organizations what lies at the core of experience success, culture is consistently the leading response. However, though most leaders may agree with these sentiments in theory, they remain uncertain about what it actually means and what it takes to get there.

Many will talk about culture in a more amorphous way. For them, good culture is a vague ideal for which they continually strive but they never quite attain. Though this conundrum has plagued leaders for decades, it has been especially pronounced over the past several years. Organizations and the people who work in them are feeling elevated pressure that makes building and sustaining culture more challenging than it ever was before.

Today, conversations regarding the importance of culture abound, yet a succinct definition remains difficult for many to grasp. As a consequence, many leaders choose to focus on the tangible, relying on actions, practices, and/or behaviors they believe will get their organization to some coveted, yet elusive, cultural ideal. To that end, an all-too-common but misinformed premise among some leaders has emerged: the simple act of doing "good" things for people, such as having coffee and a conversation with an employee or hosting a volunteer breakfast, must exemplify that an organization has a good culture.

The crucial point that these leaders miss, however, is that much more must occur *before* those practices take place. You must first choose to create a positive and personal environment and then implement defined practices to perpetuate it. Ultimately, these practices must stand on an intentionally declared and sustained strong cultural foundation. This is established through, and modeled by, leaders committed to creating environments where people thrive versus just survive. Practices implemented without this strong foundation are at risk of being unsustainable, which is why many organizations come up short in their quest for a sustained, positive culture. It's not about doing things but rather about what you *choose* to be as an organization from the outset. Leaders can implement practices all day long, but time and again they prove to be meaningless without a strong foundation on which to stand.

Successful organizations understand this. They work in significant ways to establish and support strong cultures that are built by and for the right people, framed by clear and shared expectations and values, and focused on alignment with purpose and clarity in how individual roles contribute to organizational success. They also recognize that having a strong culture grounds the patient experience they seek to provide from the very beginning. They talk about it; they breathe it; they exemplify it in every action. Culture is something people feel (and even hear about from others) long before they ever open a door to an organization.

In this way, culture acts as a bridge. It not only connects people to each other but also connects them to a common purpose. Its building blocks are composed of the shared values, mission, people, and positive interactions and experiences of an organization. A good culture is one that provides a unifying force to bridge gaps in communication, values, and perspectives. You build your culture on the people who show up to work because you've created a vibrant workforce that feels heard, engaged, and excited to be contributing to the common purpose. It's not a fluid construct; you must intentionally choose the culture you want or risk leaving it to chance. Ultimately, that is the underlying key to it all: intentional choice. In every encounter, people choose how they will interact with others. And how people interact with others, shaped by the cultures we create, is how people ultimately experience any organization.

INTENTIONAL CHOICE

As noted, creating and maintaining a strong, positive, vibrant culture is an intentional choice. It is intentionally declaring what you want to be as an organization, getting people to understand what that is, and taking action to deliver on those expectations. You build it and then sustain it based on many different ideals. As such, the answer to the question on how to achieve and sustain a great organizational culture may seem somewhat elementary. But it is that simple: intentional choice. At the same time, it is also cyclical, as culture is built on the choices that people make—and in sustaining it, positive culture will frame how people will make future choices.

This idea reaffirms that culture itself doesn't need to be created, but good culture does. Culture exists in every organization. It's analogous to the experience an individual may have with a healthcare organization. Like culture, experiences happen whether built with intention or not. Similarly, experiences, both positive and negative, stem from an initial choice. The difference is that choice can be framed and supported with intention or left to chance. However, leaving things to chance (which is still a choice) carries serious implications. A weak culture can result in negative safety, health, financial, and employee consequences. So even if you have engaged the best people, they may begin to feel defeated and ultimately leave the organization. The choices you make regarding the culture you create truly matter.

Culture is not a task to be checked off an endless to-do list; it requires consistent care and attention. Contrary to typical goal setting, without a strong and positive culture, you can never reach your ultimate goals. Consider that you would never stop watering a beautiful plant after having nurtured it to get it to a place of abundance. Culture is much the same. It takes constant watering, regardless of how good it may look at one point in time. And there is truly never a moment when you can say you've achieved great culture and declare your work done. As it relates to human experience, David Feinberg, MD, MBA, former CEO of the UCLA Hospital System and associate vice chancellor at UCLA, speaks to us about the continuing nature of this: "The minute you can tell me the person that comes next is any less important than the one we're talking to now is when we can stop." There is never a time when we can say that we have the culture and experience right and move on. It doesn't work that way.

With intentional choice, you can build the type of culture you know will deliver the experience you want to provide for your workforce, for your patients, and for your community. In doing so, you intentionally create an environment where others have the ability to make these choices—an environment where you can get the right people who make the right choices. The right choices will provide the best interactions, and the best interactions are, without doubt, what will provide the best experiences for your people, your patients, and the communities you serve.

HEALTHCARE DIFFERENTIATORS

Though the constructs in building culture are essentially the same regardless of the industry or setting, healthcare provides additional dynamics to the equation. Healthcare is unique in that it comprises human beings caring for human beings. We're not selling products or offering services. In healthcare, we are providing experiences, and when individuals engage in healthcare, either as team members or as patients, the experience they have is driven primarily by the human beings with whom they interact.

Healthcare is about the life of the person in front of you at their most vulnerable moment. No other industry truly has the same dynamic. Even in a service environment, the primary focus is on the service, not the person involved. The sheer intensity of this and the consequences involved undoubtedly impact an organization's culture, as there must be space to allow for higher emotions and critical thinking. Yet when we are intentional about allowing for this from the beginning, it will already be embedded into the culture, creating a safe place for those who need it and enabling better communication among employees, volunteers, and third parties. In that space and with better, clearer communication, patients are more likely to follow instructions, take their medications, and return for additional appointments—actions that may have life-altering consequences.

THE ROLE OF LEADERSHIP IN CULTURE

Though woven into and sustained throughout an organization, culture is primarily established with the intention and actions of leadership. For example, we've seen two hospitals in the same hospital system that have entirely different cultures. They have the same mission and the same values, so their cultures should be the same. Yet the variance in culture between the two is palpable after merely walking into each one. The difference is the result of leaders not making consistent choices to engage their people in advancing the mission and values.

At Northwell Health, they have culture influencers at the local level who are supported by experience champions and facilitators who have rolled out the organization's educational curriculum. To start, the leaders were given the opportunity to visit every site to determine who the person would be that would drive the patient experience in their specific area. The criteria were simple. They were looking for people who were role models—those who would act as change agents who could alter the status quo. And through those conversations, the leaders chose individuals to begin to lead the patient experience change at their specific site and service line. At last count, they had over 50 culture leaders across their organization ensuring that intentional choices were made daily to support and enhance their shared purpose, mission, and values.

This example shows that culture requires clear leadership that has intentional purpose, attracting the right people around a core set of values and then enforcing that purpose every day. Only then is it about the practices that are chosen to enable positive exchanges. There must be clarity around that purpose and consistency with it, including getting feedback from those who may understand it best. Support cannot be surface level. Rather, it must permeate every aspect of an organization.

Dr. Karen Grimley, chief nursing executive, UCLA Health, talks about how leaders need to show up for, and be accountable to, their people. In the past, she would ask her managers about how the employees were doing and the experience that they, and the patients, were having. Her managers told her everything they thought she wanted to hear, painting a bright picture of the employees' satisfaction and of their organizational culture. Though that may have been, on some level, what she *wanted* to hear, it wasn't what she *needed* to hear because it wasn't particularly accurate.

It wasn't until Karen went out and talked to the employees herself that she realized what was truly happening. In addition to listening, she was able to share important communications that helped the staff feel more informed and, by extension, connected to the organization. She learned that the employees had not even been aware of the important work happening within the organization that directly impacted them, including the recent addition of break relief and a med-surg transport team, among others. None of it had been communicated to the front lines.

Showing up in that way and directly offering an invitation to share openly, she was told not what she wanted to hear but what she, as a leader, needed to hear. "I knew how to fix that as the type of leader I am," she says. "You put flat shoes on and get yourself out there and see what the staff are saying." For leadership, the metrics on culture cannot be merely accepting the status quo because it's easier that way. Rather, it is taking ownership of it all—the positive and the negative. Whether it's occasional coffee chats, town halls, personal encounters on rounds, or some other practice, leaders need to show up and offer the same human touch they expect their people to provide others. When they do, incredible things will happen.

THE CHOICE TO ENGAGE OTHERS

We can understand all the data, metrics, and solutions available, but if we don't have a commitment to our employees, engaging them in how to deliver positive experiences, and we aren't clear about the expectations for what they can do to achieve that, the culture will fall short. Engagement creates the opportunity to address the challenge of employees finding themselves disconnected from the very passion and purpose that drove them to healthcare in the first place. However, engagement is about more than employees; it's also about patients and their families.

As an example, Augusta University Health, a respected institution committed to a focus on patient- and family-centered care, has 200 patient and family advisors across the organization who provide input and feedback on all aspects of the organization's efforts. Members of the team not only ask for input but also commit to acting on what they hear. This focus and committed structure, aligned with a focus on action, is a clear and extensive example of how patient and family engagement can move from concept to practice. By not just having patients and families in advisory roles but engaging them in planning and selection processes, educational efforts, and more, the organization has integrated the patient and family voice into all its operational functions.

Engagement is the result of creating vibrant and supportive cultures of service, quality, and safety. It comes from placing care at the highest order at every touch point across the continuum of care. When we choose this, we ensure the greatest of perceptions from our patients and the unparalleled experience we would want for our families and ourselves. Harvard Business School professors John Kotter and James Heskett, co-authors of the book, *Corporate Culture and Performance*, have a nice way of framing culture in the workplace at two levels: the deeper level of shared values and the visible level of shared behaviors.[24] This is the art of patient experience.

THE BENEFITS OF A STRONG CULTURE

When someone says that they do culture well in their organization, it is often a sign that they don't do it well enough. It is our experience that the organizations that tend to be high performing are the ones that think they are not doing enough or that they are never truly quite there. They understand that culture is not completed at some point in time but rather involves ongoing effort.

At the same time, a strong, vibrant, positive organizational culture will invariably attract and keep the right people as staff members, physicians, and volunteers—it will be obvious and not based on its own proclamations of "having a good culture." People want to work with and for an organization that is purposeful and supports who they are as human beings. They want to feel respected, acknowledged, and appreciated. And, of course, patients want to feel heard, cared for, and confident in a team's abilities to improve their health.

Nuria Diaz Avendaño, quality and patient experience director, Quirónsalud, reinforces the impact of turnover on patient experience: "In the summer in Spain, we notice an increase in patient safety incidents. We notice that when we have a higher turnover, less experienced people, our patients suffer."

In an effort to better see what getting it right resembles, we interviewed leaders from VHA's Patient Experience Office, exploring their efforts to transform organizational culture and rebuild trust with veteran patients. As the largest U.S. integrated healthcare system, VHA serves 9 million veterans across 1,293 facilities.[25] The Veterans Experience Office strives to enhance both patient experience and trust to combat an ongoing image problem.

VHA defined its patient experience, adopted a human-centered design, and implemented "The Voice of the Veteran" program. Then, benchmarking against best practices, it developed tool kits and the PX Road Map to Excellence, guiding an enterprise-wide, action-oriented approach to elevate patient experience.[26]

In only a five-year span, VHA's efforts yielded impressive results. Its patient experience had matched or exceeded that of private-sector healthcare systems in quality, outperforming in 10 out of 11 metrics. Trust scores surged by 24 percent, and over 54 percent of VHA Health Systems achieved a top-tier rating on HCAHPS survey. Addressing employee engagement challenges, VHA now ranks fifth among federal agencies, showcasing a substantial improvement in delivering exceptional customer experiences.

In the *To Care Is Human* podcast, Jennifer Purdy, executive director CX tools and implementation, Department of Veterans Affairs, talks specifically about this sweet spot: "Where the magic really happens is being able to find a way to connect to the employee to allow them to see that what they do every day matters. They're part of something bigger than themselves. We can create solutions, even small ones, but having that feeling and allowing that to perpetuate and propel the staff and movement of employees, that's where the magic happens. In essence, that is the human experience."[27]

What VHA did fundamentally revolved around the power of choice. It prioritized the experience first. Comprehending its significance, it then actively chose to embody it in its practices. The VHA team measured results and adjusted where necessary—and the results speak for themselves.

There is a remarkable return on investment for intentionally choosing to create and maintain a great culture. The transformative impact of a consciously chosen and nurtured culture is evident in the holistic well-being of an organization, and the ripple effects are far-reaching. In contrast, in situations where leadership has not made the intentional choice and commitment to create and foster a positive culture, the impacts are just as palpable. An atmosphere of indifference prevails and is obvious to both employees and patients. They can feel it the moment they walk through the door.

The absence of a strong, positive culture also creates additional challenges in healthcare, where most individuals are drawn to working in the industry by a sense of purpose larger than themselves. Neglecting this purpose with a poor culture erodes morale, leading to considerable troubles. Every choice made carries consequences, either positive or negative, underscoring the crucial link between intentionality and the far-reaching implications that reverberate across various aspects of an organization.

ESTABLISHING AND REINFORCING A STRONG, VIBRANT, AND POSITIVE ORGANIZATIONAL CULTURE

Any time choices are as paramount as they are to culture, accountability is a factor. Accountability is the backbone of a robust culture. It ensures that individuals take ownership of their choices and actions and that they align with shared values while contributing to a positive work environment. Accountability helps foster transparency, trust, and a sense of ownership among a team to shape a culture of excellence.

Building a basis for accountability in culture requires creating ownership around several committed actions, without which organizations run the risk of falling short on their defined culture and, by extension, patient experience objectives. They include the following:

1. **Establish focused standards/expectations.** Determine and clearly define what you expect in terms of behaviors and actions as you create a culture of accountability.
2. **Set clear consequences for inaction and rewards and recognition for action.** Be willing to reinforce expectations consistently and use them as opportunities for learning.
3. **Provide learning opportunities to understand and see expectations in action.** Ensure that staff at all levels are clear on expected behaviors and consequences.
4. **Communicate expectations, reinforcing what and why consistently and continuously.** Keep expectations top of mind and be clear that they are part of what you are as an organization in every encounter.
5. **Observe and evaluate staff at all levels, providing feedback and/or coaching as needed.** Turn actual encounters, good or bad, into learning moments and opportunities to ensure that people are clear on expected behaviors and actions.
6. **Execute on consequences immediately and thoughtfully.** Respond rapidly when people miss the mark (or when people excel) to ensure that people are aware of the importance of your expectations.
7. **Revisit expectations often to ensure that they meet the needs and objectives of the organization.** Remember that standards and expectations are dynamic and change with your organization's needs. They must stay in tune with what you are as an organization (your values) and where you intend to go (your vision).

Through all our research and explorations at The Beryl Institute into what drives the best in experience, there has always been an element of these simple organizational truths, which represent creating ownership of a culture that prioritizes experience. Simply putting tactics in place runs the risk of turning your patient experience efforts into the latest "flavor of the month" activity. Patients and their families, as well as your colleagues and employees, deserve much more. To truly drive an exceptional patient experience, you can only influence perceptions through the choices you make—one of the most critical of those being the type of organizational culture you choose to create.

To truly drive an exceptional patient experience, you can only influence perceptions through the choices you make—one of the most critical of those being the type of organizational culture you choose to create.

Culture is a comprehensive and continuous approach that is perpetual in the support shown to others. It is actively listening to patients and their families, showing empathy, and taking actions that align with your values and mission to truly foster community well-being around you. At the highest level, and at the heart of it all, is the capacity not only to make choices but also to make better choices. Effective solutions stem from consistently making these sound decisions. Choose to have a good culture. Choose to have positive interaction. Choose to care for your workforce. Choose to prioritize human experience and all that it entails. This rests on the intentionality of those who are in positions to make these choices. Though tactics and best practices play a role, your intentional choice to cultivate a positive culture will stand out as the most influential factor in shaping a consistently positive and impactful human experience.

What Is the Impact?

- Increased workplace safety
- Sustained high reliability
- Boosted external ratings

CHAPTER 5

People Are the Primary Drivers of Experience

Guiding Principle: Understand and act on the needs and vulnerabilities of the healthcare workforce

Key Takeaways

1. The healthcare workforce is the primary conduit through which any experience is delivered.
2. Organizations must support and care for their workforce in order to foster engagement, wellness, and growth.
3. Active engagement of the healthcare workforce is vital and involves not just listening to their concerns but also taking meaningful actions based on their feedback.

This chapter, building on the importance of culture as a foundation for any experience effort, affirms that if we are to provide excellence in experience, organizations must strive to understand, meet the needs of, and actively engage the voices of those who work in healthcare every day. This concept dives deep into the notion that healthcare organizations must support and care for their workforce in order to foster engagement, wellness, and growth. The reason that this is so crucial to success in delivering exceptional experience is that it is the people in any healthcare organization who are the primary conduit through which that experience is delivered. Caring for them and engaging them as the owners of the experience is a critical way to deliver on it.

This requires organizations to work to intentionally understand and act on the needs of those showing up to work every day. Rick Evans, SVP and CXO, New York-Presbyterian Hospital, speaks of this link: "I've learned throughout my career, mostly from my mistakes, quite frankly, that you really can't ask anyone to do something for patient experience if you can't also answer, 'What's in it for the employee? What can really make their experience better?'"[28]

This topic is also inextricably linked with the importance of organizational culture that we explored in Chapter 4. Though there is a clear link from culture to people, what we are considering now is what happens *after* you have the right people who are helping to intentionally perpetuate the right culture. Establishing clear expectations and facilitating effective engagement with them requires the same level of intentionality as cultivating culture. In fact, it's rooted in the same premise as humanity itself—creating environments that individuals are not only attracted to but also where they desire to remain. When you connect culture to people and vice versa, the lines between them inevitably blur. The people in an organization reflect its culture, and the culture is perpetuated through the actions of its people. The question that is left is, "How do you care for them so that they'll not only physically stay but also remain committed to sustaining that culture? And even more importantly, a culture of experience excellence?"

HEALTHCARE FACTORS

When discussing individuals within a healthcare organization's workforce, whether they are physicians, employees, volunteers, or contracted staff, we are not drawing distinctions about who works for whom. Though we recognize that not every individual, such as certain physicians, may be directly employed by an organization, and that different roles entail different needs, it's crucial to provide support to *all* individuals contributing to a healthcare environment. Even the term "workforce" in and of itself can be problematic. For our purposes, we're referring to the people within your organization who collectively shape its culture and deliver the desired experience.

Ultimately, everyone shares the responsibility for steering the organization in the same direction.

We would also be remiss not to acknowledge that those working in healthcare today are under a continuous amount of stress. Healthcare has become a complex, dynamic, and even chaotic system that puts tremendous pressure on the workforce to balance navigating process and providing high levels of compassionate care. With the very nature of healthcare itself—as we shared earlier, as human beings caring for human beings—emotions can run high in nearly every interaction with patients, families, and coworkers. Your people need a safe space to debrief and effectively deal with not only these emotional impacts but also the consequential burnout, which, despite increased attention recently, has been problematic for decades. We have been talking about burnout for decades, but these discussions were exacerbated by the pandemic, when our veneers were pulled back, truly revealing the daily challenges faced by healthcare professionals.

If we are remiss in acknowledging and acting on this current reality, people are apt to leave their organizations. In fact, many already have. A report from the U.S. Labor Department revealed that more than half a million healthcare workers quit their jobs in August 2021, nearly a 20-percent increase from the 404,000 resignations recorded a year prior.[29] These findings further revealed that nurses were at greater risk than ever as they tackled the pandemic, natural disasters, conflicts, and political upheaval.

Annette Kennedy, president of the International Council of Nurses, describes the current environment relevant to nurses practicing around the globe by stating, "Our nurses, your nurses, need to be taken care of so that they can keep returning to work every day and do their unique work of helping to keep patients and families safe and well."[30]

Once again, we must circle back to culture. Those who work in healthcare tend to arrive with purpose and passion. Caring for others, in any respect, is a true calling. What you choose to do in your organization—in your culture—can either kindle that flame or douse it. Kindling creates an environment that will fuel that passion even further. Alina Moran, president and CEO of Dignity Health California Hospital Medical Center, speaks of an experience survey they conducted with their staff: "One of the things that we always score high on is that they find their work meaningful, that they live our mission each and every day, that the patients they serve are so important to them. It's all about those human-to-human relationships, and it comes back to knowing that those relationships are saving and changing lives and reducing human suffering." This connection to meaning and purpose, and the intentional effort to continually foster a sense of purpose and passion, are essential to caring for your workforce and ensuring excellence in experience.

ENGAGING VOICES

As the guiding principle sets forth, this starts by understanding the needs of and engaging the voices of your people. Engagement, however, must be looked at as the comprehensive term it is—one that extends beyond mere acknowledgment. Engagement is actively listening to employees, understanding their concerns, and addressing their needs. We need to care for them, not just passively hear their words. Though ensuring that they feel heard is important, simply listening without taking action or demonstrating a genuine concern renders the effort meaningless. What matters most is what happens next in how that input is used to drive tangible outcomes and improvements. The real value lies in what follows: taking action and driving meaningful change.

Jim Dunn, president and CEO of LD Human Capital Consulting and former executive vice president and enterprise chief people and culture officer at Atrium Health, shares the success of shifting the annual employee engagement survey to anniversary surveys: "Every day, we push out between 3 and 500 surveys and get real-time feedback. People's needs are immediate. For example, if an employee needs childcare today, you can't capture that on a survey in four or five months. That person will probably have gone somewhere that provides childcare."

It's not merely effectuating change on leadership's part, though. Individuals need to feel empowered to take action themselves, which requires actively framing opportunities for them to contribute and make a difference. It's important to understand your team's needs and priorities, as they are the ones who possess invaluable insights and ideas. Failure to involve the voices of your team generally doesn't bode well. Consider the cautionary tale of a hospital that, despite its intention to create the best ER in the country, neglected to involve ER staff in the design process. As a result, the new facility proved impractical and challenging to work in, highlighting the importance of incorporating frontline perspectives in this type of decision-making.

In contrast, Dr. Teresa Anderson, chief executive at Sydney Local Health District in Australia, directly involved her staff in developing a model of patient and family-centered care—not because she had to, per se, but rather because she knew that she needed their input:

> That included our policies and procedures but also how we orient our staff, how we select our staff, and

what decisions we make that truly support patient and family-centered care. Our staff was always a key part of that, and it wasn't just about educating them in patient- and family-centered care. It was really about, "How do we create an environment that enables our staff to provide patient and family-centered care and excellent clinical care?" That's about supporting the staff, providing an environment that is enriching for them, supporting their professional development, and making them feel really good when they come to work so that they can have those conversations with our patients in a positive way. It was also about our environments, including our physical environments for both our staff and our patients. We want staff who are happy and feel fulfilled.

What matters most in engaging people's voices is ensuring that everyone feels heard, safe, engaged, and supported. At its core, this is about addressing the fundamental human needs of those working in healthcare. It's about prioritizing the basics. Only then can those voices be used to help drive comprehensive and lasting solutions.

DRIVING COMPREHENSIVE AND LASTING SOLUTIONS

We put leaders in place, create a good culture, and use that culture to attract and retain the best people. It is critical that organizations then invest with intention to support them. In many cases, the solutions that must be developed are centered on sustaining well-being. As previously discussed, those who work in healthcare operate in a stressful environment simply by the nature of their job. A broader perspective that includes holistic well-being is one vital piece in addressing that stress.

Though well-being starts with an individual's basic health, attention to it requires oversight from professionals. For example, some organizations have brought licensed social workers onboard to offer coaching or counseling sessions with employees, while one organization expanded its employee assistance program (EAP) to cover all three shifts at each location across its system. Still another embedded trained peer counselors inside each of its units. Given the importance of diet and nutrition on overall health and wellness, other organizations have developed programs that address the role of diet on emotional wellness by providing employees with access to a nutritionist.

Organizations such as these, the ones that understand the importance of this premise, make a commitment to creating and implementing solutions that extend beyond simply telling their people that *they care*. More importantly, they show them through the actions they take. And though these actions and the examples we share that follow are critical, there also needs to be a fundamental commitment from organizations that they create a space where it is okay not to be okay—spaces where being stressed or burned out is not seen as a negative reflection on an individual but rather as a consequence of the realities of healthcare, which can often perpetuate these feelings. When we support people in realizing that the way they feel isn't bad but instead is simply a reality that all are committed to addressing, we make great strides in creating environments of well-being. It is the actions we take and the space we give people that matter most.

The following are a sampling of these types of actions, common practices that organizations have used to demonstrate how they listen to, recognize, and engage their people:

Team Lavender

As the world continued to take inventory of the wake left by the COVID-19 pandemic, healthcare organizations and leaders remained steadfast and focused on recovery. At Northwell Health, the largest health system in New York State, employee emotional wellness remained a constant priority. Team Lavender (TL) was developed as an interdisciplinary group of professionals dedicated to supporting colleagues during times of stress and/or hardship. Emergent and proactive TL peer support responses/activations provided a moment of pause, reflection, teamwork, and peer support—and then it grew from there.

Agnes Barden, vice president, Office of Patient and Customer Experience at Northwell Health, notes how this intentional action had a ripple effect: "TL came from the innate need of individuals who want to truly care for each other's well-being and subsequently has taken on this major ripple effect across our organization. What started at one hospital quickly spread throughout the organization."[31]

This solution addressed the need to leverage the power of peer support during an exceedingly difficult time. These individuals would go home to their family and friends and try to explain what they had seen, what they had gone through. And though their loved ones may have listened and empathized, they could not fully understand, through no fault of their own.

These healthcare workers are humans caring for other humans, and there is something really unique, hard, and beautiful about that responsibility. As such, TL has bloomed over the years because of its simplicity. That is, there are no algorithms, checklists, or metrics; rather, it's about human needs. At the core of TL is having a colleague truly see you, hear you, and be still with you for a moment of time.

Code Lavender

Similar to Northwell, managers at ECU Health in North Carolina needed a one-stop shop to be able to find organizational well-being resources. Though they had developed many offerings for their team members, the Office of Wellbeing thought it would be helpful to house them under one umbrella to better serve the workforce. The action they took was adopting Code Lavender as a holistic care response framework to assist healthcare teams in need of well-being support during times of increased emotional stress or after a distressing event.

The framework consisted of 12 support mechanisms offering individualized approaches for care teams. Offerings included Lavender Rounds, Critical Incident Response, Listening Circles, Wellbeing Rounds, Wellbeing Pop-ups, Team Building and Professional Development, MD/APP Peer Support, Caring for the Caregiver Peer Support, Office of Experience, Customized Wellbeing Workshops, Spiritual Support, and Workplace Aggression Reporting.

This framework allowed ECU Health to individualize offerings to meet the team's needs. They noted that it is often used when managers reach out and say, "I am not sure what our team needs." They simply call a Code Lavender and are then assisted in customized interventions. They have found this to be an excellent way for teams to see on one page all the available resources. This availability results in increased use, as shown by the following outcomes:

- Forty percent increase in EAP utilization
- Improved team member resilience index from 46th to 63rd percentile ranking related to team members' ability to decompress and disconnect from work
- Improved physician overall alignment and engagement post-three-day well-being workshop

Leadership Rounding

Leadership rounding has proven to be an effective solution to issues regarding engagement with those in healthcare. When department directors, VPs, senior administrators, and supervisors walk around to talk to others and spend time on the floor, it lets the team know they care about them by both literally and figuratively meeting them where they are. From the leaders' perspective, rounding helps them understand the pain points of their employees and how to bring solutions to their daily work.

Regularly checking in with employees in this way to inquire about how they can better support them should be a standard practice throughout any organization and irrespective of individual roles. Rick Evans, SVP and CXO, New York-Presbyterian Hospital, speaks of this inclusivity: "At NYP, every person in every role counts. We will treat everyone as valued human beings, considering his or her feelings, needs, ideas, and preferences. We will honor everyone's contributions to creating a healing environment for our patients and families."[32]

This inclusive approach ensures that every member of the team feels valued and empowered to voice their needs and concerns. By soliciting feedback from employees at all levels, organizations can gain a comprehensive understanding of the support mechanisms required to nurture a positive work environment and promote employee well-being. This proactive approach not only demonstrates a commitment to employee satisfaction and growth but also facilitates the identification of systemic issues and opportunities for improvement that may otherwise go unnoticed.

Schwartz Center Rounds

The Schwartz Center Rounds program offers healthcare providers a regularly scheduled time to openly and honestly discuss the social and emotional issues they face in caring for patients and families. This program now takes place in more than 425 healthcare organizations throughout the United States, Canada, Australia, and New Zealand and more than 150 sites throughout the United Kingdom and Ireland. In contrast to traditional medical rounds, the focus is on the human dimension of medicine. Panelists from diverse disciplines, including physicians, nurses, social workers, psychologists, allied health professionals, and chaplains, as well as anyone who is part of the overall patient experience, including security and even parking staff and environmental services, participate in the sessions. Caregivers then have an opportunity to share their experiences, thoughts, and feelings on thought-provoking topics drawn from these actual patient cases.

Caregivers who've participated in multiple Schwartz Center Rounds sessions have reported the following:

- Increased insight into the social and emotional aspects of patient care, increased feelings of compassion, and increased readiness to respond to patients' and families' needs
- Improved teamwork, interdisciplinary communication, and appreciation for the roles and contributions of colleagues from different disciplines
- Decreased feelings of stress and isolation and more openness to giving and receiving support

In many cases, participants have reported that insights gained during Schwartz Center Rounds led to the implementation of specific changes in departmental or hospital-wide practices or policies to benefit both patients and providers.[33]

Soul Snacks

"Soul Snack LIVE!" presentations were developed as virtual peer-to-peer staff support programs to promote spiritual and emotional wellness among healthcare staff at Kaiser Permanente's Marin/Sonoma Service Area in Northern California. Provided by its Spiritual Care Services Department, the "Snacks" are 15-minute offerings presented monthly by staff members who play many different roles across various departments and disciplines at Kaiser's facilities. Drawing from personal experience, they share with fellow colleagues their own unique answers to the question, "How do you tend to your spiritual and emotional well-being, especially in the midst of our stressful work?"[34]

The topics cover a vast range of healing modalities, from meditation to music, painting to humming, self-compassion to healing laughter, relaxation to marathon running. The result has been what Karen Hulsey, MSN, RN, Kaiser Permanente continuum administrator at Marin/Sonoma, describes as a domino effect that has created a culture shift throughout the facilities:

> We've had physician chiefs do soul snacks; we've had EVS workers do soul snacks...When you hear somebody say, "I do struggle, and the way I get through the day is by writing a poem or singing a song or visualizing something," you go, "Oh, so I can be a whole person? I can be a person who is successful and who is competent and a person who struggles and has to cope with it?" And in fact, that ripple effect of acknowledgment is going to knit me together with all of the people I work with.[35]

At the heart of all the above-mentioned examples is ensuring that people feel heard and cared for—not merely so they can do their job but holistically to truly ensure their well-being and demonstrate that someone in the organization cares. These practices are merely some of many that help to create a place where people not only want to come to work but also will tell others to join them. Other considerations in driving solutions include the following:

- Including well-being in strategic and financial planning
- Focusing on crisis prevention while also knowing the signals of burnout and acting quickly
- Placing well-being support programs at the core of business operations
- Creating a culture of wellness through education

- Encouraging tactics that help staff with balancing professional and personal priorities
- Recognizing, rewarding, and celebrating people

RECOGNITION AND CELEBRATION

Recognition is a powerful tool that can impact many of these solutions we've discussed. It has been shown to bolster the engagement of staff, increase satisfaction, and even boost motivation. Yet we suggest taking one more step beyond acknowledgement and recognition to where a magical opportunity we often fall short of in healthcare exists: the power of celebration.

This is beyond the surface of hanging a sign on a unit to say congratulations for a performance achievement or even singing "Happy Birthday" at monthly staff forums. Though we can agree that these activities are part of creating cultures of engagement, they are more representative of simple and thoughtful acknowledgement of accomplishment, not the true sense of celebration. By "celebration," we are talking about deeper acknowledgement and the emotional connection that we have to our success. Celebration is not simply a certificate or a banner. It is the true expression of appreciation from the heart—one shared with colleagues and peers. Celebration, from this perspective, is an experience itself.

Using celebration in this regard may be the attendance of a senior leader at a unit huddle to express why the service efforts of a staff member had a positive impact on the experience of a patient or family member. It could be bringing the prom or an anniversary or birthday party to a patient's room. It could be a red-carpet welcome in the lobby for a volunteer on the

> *Recognition is something you do; it is rational and thoughtful. Celebration is something you experience; it is emotional and heartfelt.*

day that marks her 20 years of service or a thoughtful send-off for a long-time patient who healed and is now leaving your facility. Once practiced, the difference between celebrating and recognizing is almost tangible. You feel it on the inside. Recognition is something you do; it is rational and thoughtful. Celebration is something you experience; it is emotional and heartfelt.

In a work environment where stress can run high and emotion sits just below (and at times above) the surface in every encounter, by moving beyond recognition (not leaving it behind) and ensuring true celebration, we intentionally provide an experience for our team, our patients, our families, and our communities. The reality is that they are having an experience whether we design one or not. In celebration, we create lasting memories, the very essence of experience itself—that which is remembered. In doing so, we unleash the potential of our people, acknowledge the humanity of our patients, and allow the true purpose and passion in our work to emerge. Through celebration, we enliven and enrich our organizations and create new opportunities to positively impact the patient experience through stronger relationships.

IMPORTANCE OF RELATIONSHIPS AND BUILDING TRUST

Underlying every aspect of the guiding principle highlighted in this chapter is a foundation built on relationships. We simply cannot engage others' voices or support them in order to drive comprehensive solutions without having a strong relationship first. Dr. Harish Pillai, group CEO at Metro Pacific Health, speaks about the broader impact of the real return on value for investing in a focus on human experience:

> This is all to do with people experiences. I have seen in my own experience in different organizations that when you invest in relationships with your staff, that

staff has got an X factor because they go beyond the call of service to ensure that at every episodic encounter there's a "wow" feeling. They exceed expectations. You can only have such motivated staff when they themselves feel empowered and happy in an organization because it's not a salary which motivates. It's that kind of an empowering environment. And autonomy of function, especially for healthcare workers—I think that's critical because traditionally we are very hierarchical. But even within a certain hierarchy, if you can give functional autonomy, it actually empowers quite a bit to healthcare workers, and that can result in such kind of superlative experiences.

One underlying component of these relationships is trust. Our capacity for trust in ourselves and others determines how we respond to situations where threats, conflict, or controversy arise. Knowing ourselves, what we stand for in life and work, our own unique histories with trust, and our response patterns provides the foundation for trusting relationships with others, including patients, families, colleagues, leaders, and the broader society.

Previous experiences may have eroded our capacity to trust ourselves, each other, and the systems where we work and, in some measure, the surrounding communities and societal structures in which we live. In these cases, a pathway to foster healing relationships must be forged. To ultimately address specific challenges, including how best to balance patient/family experience with staff safety and well-being, The Beryl Institute's Nurse Executive Council coalesced around a framework of healing as a path to rebuild trust after the pandemic. This involved the application of skills associated with trauma-informed care, including the proposed steps for healing when trust is broken—shifting from a sense of despair to a hopeful future.

There will inevitably be moments when trust has either been fostered or broken. Depending on the perspective, these instances most likely have accumulated, impacting our well-being and that of others. According to the Reina Trust Model framework, a model illustrating the important components that contribute to trust between people, within teams, and throughout organizations, "Ninety percent of behaviors that break trust in workplace relationships are small, subtle, and unintentional."[36] Trust rebuilding includes the following:

- **Trust of character.** This begins with being a person who can be relied and depended on. It requires a belief in mutually serving intentions and is strengthened by managing expectations, having clear boundaries, showing consistency in behavior, keeping promises and agreements, and delegating responsibly.
- **Trust of communication.** This relies on openly, honestly, and transparently sharing information, admitting and taking responsibility for missteps or mistakes, giving and receiving feedback in a respectful manner, upholding confidentiality, and speaking in a manner that reflects self-respect and respect of others.
- **Trust of capability.** This is built when an individual knows and honors their own skills, abilities, and limitations while concomitantly recognizing the capabilities of others, expresses appreciation for the contributions of others, involves people in decision-making, and encourages an environment of learning.

Using the Reina Trust Model as a foundation, the group generated tangible steps to be considered in association with components of building trust, which included the following:

- Invest in basic human needs.
- Intensify human connection.

- Create open spaces for listening (without fixing whatever is shared).
- Begin the healing process (by acknowledging what has happened previously).
- Take responsibility for the decisions that were made and, when needed, admit missteps and make amends that are meaningful to the people impacted by them.
- Move from transactional to relational communication.
- Invite thoughtful input.
- Dissolve silos.
- Commit to transforming human experience in healthcare.

Your people serve as the backbone of your healthcare delivery system and, in essence, are the foundation of the overall experience you provide. They are the ones who translate your promises into reality—whether it's the assurance of quality care in the surgery suite or the commitment to excellent service when addressing patient inquiries about billing. Getting these fundamentals right is paramount to success. In fact, when you get this right, it accounts for a vast majority of that success. Everything else—your strategies, policies, and procedures—are at great risk if your people are not engaged and cannot effectively execute on them.

> *Your people serve as the backbone of your healthcare delivery system and, in essence, are the foundation of the overall experience you provide. They are the ones who translate your promises into reality.*

Nicole Cable, former chief experience officer, CareMax, reinforces the opportunity by having team members actively engaged in experience efforts: "Your people have to believe it's not just lip service. Then they'll be your champions. They will stay loyal to you. They will tell their friends and family about you. If people on social media are throwing you under the bus, they will jump in and defend you. You don't have to say anything because they will have your back. But if you are not focused on human experience and truly taking care of people and doing what's right by them, you are never going to get to the next level."

This means not only hearing your employees' words but actively listening to their meaning, caring for their well-being, and acting on their needs and vulnerabilities to honor their commitment and reaffirm their purpose. It's about providing the support and development opportunities they need to excel while fostering a sense of ownership in their ability to fulfill their roles effectively. By setting the right expectations, offering meaningful support, and taking effective action, you're empowering them to deliver on your organization's mission with excellence.

What Is the Impact?

- Improved workforce engagement
- Elevated team member attraction/retention
- Enhanced workforce well-being

CHAPTER 6

Engaging Patient and Care Partners Is a Must

Guiding Principle: Implement a defined process for formal, intentional, and continuous partnerships with patients, families, and care partners

Key Takeaways
1. Patients and care partners must be both intentionally and actively engaged as co-designers in the care process and included as key members of their care team.
2. Healthcare organizations must understand and address what matters most to patients and their care partners and ensure that their voices are integral in the decision-making process.
3. Formal partnership roles for patients and care partners should be established to ensure active participation in the design and improvement of healthcare services overall.

We cannot and must not have a conversation about patient experience without also discussing how we include, engage, and partner with patients. The very idea of patients at the center of this conversation is the cornerstone of the evolution of patient experience itself. From patients' rights and advocacy to overall service excellence, determining that which matters most to the people whom healthcare serves has ultimately been essential to providing positive health outcomes. And we acknowledge that the patient's perspective remains an opportunity for organizations to better focus on with clear intention to this day.

Patients and care partners, which can include family members, friends, and others whom the patient identifies as important to them in their care process, bring a unique and invaluable perspective not only to the barriers and gaps faced across the healthcare system

> *Patients are the primary experts on themselves and their lived experience—the insights, perspectives, and more—that they bring with them into a healthcare experience.*

but also to the solutions required to ensure excellence. More importantly, patients are the primary experts on themselves and their lived experience—the insights, perspectives, and more—that they bring with them into a healthcare experience. The lived experience is unique to each individual and shapes who they are and how they engage in healthcare. It ultimately frames what matters to them as an individual beyond just the clinical practice of care. This recognition enables healthcare organizations to care for the whole person who seeks their help. This is highlighted in the "Declaration for Human Experience," where one of the four commitments calls for us to "recognize and maintain a focus on what matters most to patients, their family members, and care partners to ensure unparalleled care and a commitment to health and wellbeing."[37]

Healthcare organizations generally understand that involving patients and care partners is something they should do. Some will ask patients questions about their experience when they are being discharged. Many will form an advisory council or perhaps occasionally send out a survey. Though each of these acts is flooded with good intentions, alone, they fall short, risking a decrease in the trust of patients and care partners and, consequently, a decrease in overall healthcare outcomes.

A road map for action starts by redefining and advancing the integrated nature of, and critical role that patients and their care partners play on care teams, in the following ways:

We must be intentional in redefining what we mean by "care team" to ensure the inclusion of the patient's and care partner's voices. Critical actions include the following:

- Identifying care team members, including the patient's family, healthcare providers, and the patient's circle of support
- Orienting care team members, including the patient, to their roles, responsibilities, and benefits of being an active part of the care team
- Including a formal care partner as part of the patient's care team and considering peer mentors and cultural brokers and partners

We must be consistent in inviting and activating partnership to ensure the best outcomes for patients. Critical actions include the following:

- Ensuring that patients and families co-develop the care plan and are an active part of care team interactions and decision-making discussions
- Identifying and acting on what matters most to patients, families, and each patient's circle of support
- Identifying and eliminating barriers to effective care team partnership
- Encouraging patients and families to serve in roles beyond their own care journey[38]

The commitment to engaging patient and care partner voices must start at the top with healthcare leadership in order to re-affirm commitment and address budgetary and infrastructure requirements. As organizations consider the range of possible methods of engagement, they must commit to having the infrastructure in place to support increased engagement at multiple levels. Engagement of patient voice then can be considered and implemented in a variety of ways, from individuals in their own or a loved one's care experience to formal structures such as councils within the broader healthcare organization to strategic roles as co-designers and active participants in other strategic efforts. We explore the opportunities and implications of these commitments below.

PARTNERING IN CARE

Approaching this process deliberately requires organizations to consider what intentionality entails in practice when we are partnering in care with patients and care partners. Understanding that various approaches can be utilized, the emphasis lies in actively engaging their voices. This engagement involves how organizations interact with patients, families, and care partners who are currently in the care process. It includes not only asking them how well their expectations were met at discharge but also, and more importantly, asking them when they first arrive about what those expectations are. After all, how can we know what matters most to them if we never ask? This simple act can significantly enhance their experience and preemptively address potential issues—even if their response is that they don't really care.

Intentionally engaging the voices of both patients and care partners is based on understanding what is most important to them. We cannot assume that each individual who walks in the door actually wishes to actively engage with the healthcare organization as a partner or that our patient experience strategy should be exactly the same for everyone—it won't be. Some people will prefer to be engaged participants, while others would rather see a less active approach. Understanding these differences is a skill that requires keen observation and empathy as well as the commitment to ask what matters to people.

If patients and care partners do not want to be involved as active partners, then that is their expectation. That is their chosen experience, and we must respect it. We shouldn't force them because we feel that "it's the right thing to do." Their perception is the reality regardless of what that perception may be. It is their lived experience that matters most, not what we think it should be.

Our approach must revolve around discovering how they prefer to engage in their healthcare journey. Pressing individuals into a partnership model against their wishes simply because it aligns with a perceived ideal is actually counter to providing excellence in experience. Respect for patient voice means honoring their decisions, even if they differ from our own preconceived notions of what the "best" approach is. This is about personalized care—and is a model that most healthcare organizations are moving toward.

One of the results of providing this type of personalized care is that it will inspire more individuals to participate in the experience in ways that matter to them, with outcomes that are much different than for those without personalization. With a focus on personalized care, a commitment to understanding preferences and engaging

> *With a focus on personalized care, a commitment to understanding preferences and engaging people's lived experience, people feel heard and engaged as participants and co-designers of their own care.*

people's lived experience, people feel heard and engaged as participants and co-designers of their own care.

Tony Serge, co-chair of The Beryl Institute's Global Patient and Family Advisory Board, a senior patient and family advisor (PFA) and past co-chair for multiple PFAC organizations in Massachusetts, noted a personalized care experience where, at every visit, it seemed as though an extraordinarily busy oncologist and team had only one patient: Tony's wife. "They always figured it out," he says. "No matter how busy they were, as a patient and a care partner, we never felt rushed, unheard, or undervalued. That's the level of personalization that was involved, and that personalized care inspired me to ask, 'How can I give back?'"

On the path of providing personalized care, organizations tend to get stuck on how to offer it in a scalable way. Yet engaging the voices of patients and care partners is the very vehicle to do so. You can only offer personalized care by being clear and listening to what matters most to them. In a recent interview, Marie Judd, national vice president, consumer experience at Ascension, addresses this very point:

> We talked a lot about the concept of what matters most to that person and embedding it in all of our different listening posts, whether it was through rounding or conversations that we were having with care teams, patients, and families. What we heard was really interesting—it was everything from "I want to be able to do this hike with my grandkids post X, Y, Z procedure" [to] "I want to make sure that I live for the next two years to go to my daughter's wedding" [to] "I want to be able to eat ice cream." We heard that a lot in our senior-living facility. "You know what matters most to me? I want to have a treat every night," whatever that is. It was really interesting when we started more intentionally listening for beyond the care plan and how not clinical focused it was oftentimes, and how we were able to meet more

of those human needs. "It's really important to me that you update my wife every hour while I'm in this procedure," whatever that was. How do we make sure that we attend to what matters most for that person?

Embracing the lived experience of each individual is fundamental to fostering a patient-centered approach within healthcare. By understanding their needs and wants proactively, we can ascertain whether they desire and wish to engage in a collaborative partnership. However, this dialogue often remains untapped for several reasons.

Doctors and others working in healthcare are extremely busy. As such, a number of people in these positions identify this lack of time as a rationale for why they cannot engage with patients and care partners regarding their expectations. This perspective overlooks the clear impact that this intentional (and minimal) investment in effort can have. The mere seconds invested in these conversations yield substantial savings in time, resources, and finances over the long term and lead to better outcomes overall.

Additionally, others may come from a place where they feel that they don't need feedback from patients and care partners because they are the experts on the care they provide. Though clinicians undeniably possess expertise in diagnoses and treatments, it is equally important to recognize that patients are the foremost authorities on their own experiences and preferences. Bridging these time and expertise gaps necessitates a middle ground where varying perspectives can converge to improve outcomes.

FORMAL PARTNERSHIPS

Parallel to partnering with patients and care partners around someone's individual encounter, there has also been an intentional commitment in many healthcare organizations to ensure partnership beyond the patient's own care journey. One way to activate this partnership by more formal means is by serving as a PFA. This role is intended for patients and family members, or care partners who engage with a healthcare system more strategically, to provide input and insights and broader feedback based on both their personal expertise and lived experience. PFAs serve as pivotal guides as healthcare organizations strive not only to do what is good for their own organizational operations but ultimately to ensure that they do what is best for the people they serve.

Libby Hoy, founder and CEO of PFCCpartners, a network of over 800 patient and family advisors, notes, "Patient and family caregiver engagement is not something to be sprinkled on a cake after it is baked." Hoy approaches her work in an integrated, collaborative, and partnering way but through a quality lens. "Too often," she says, "hospitals tend to think of patient and family partners 'helping' with patient experience efforts when, more importantly, they should be 'informing' not only experience but also the hospital's patient safety and quality goals."[39] As Hoy asserts, and we believe, PFAs are and should be engaged as strategic partners in the broadest sense as healthcare organizations strive to meet their experience and overall objectives.

The successful engagement of PFAs depends, however, on an organization's holistic embrace of them as partners and critical resources in support of overall success. This holistic embrace is the essence of both the guiding principle and the commitments to transforming human experience. It pertains to organizational ethos and how an organization wants to position itself on an ongoing basis, notwithstanding a specific patient outcome. It is important that healthcare organizations intentionally ensure that patients and care partners are seen as strategic partners in what the organizations do. It is not merely inviting people to be a PFA or to sit on a council as a "check-the-box" activity to say you have patient advisors; rather, it is a commitment to activating that partnership in meaningful ways.

Many individuals, such as community members, former patients, or care partners, who aren't currently active patients, are brought in to be involved in councils or other advisory roles, bringing valuable experience and a desire to contribute to improvement efforts overall. One of the most common methods for doing so is by establishing a patient and family advisory council (PFAC) to provide a structured platform for input from those directly impacted by healthcare services.

First introduced in the late 1990s, more than 2,000 hospitals now use PFACs. In fact, in some states, such as Massachusetts, PFACs are mandated. Yet as of 2021, only 51 percent of the nation's hospitals had implemented and operationalized PFACs.[40] Generally, PFACs are composed of 5 to 20 patients and care partners who meet periodically with hospital staff to provide feedback and input on a wide range of issues, including improving patient experience, increasing safety, and enhancing the quality of care.

There is ample evidence that formally and proactively inviting PFAs to guide, and even co-design, healthcare experiences is essential for tackling some of healthcare's most difficult challenges.[41] Those who understand the value of PFACs find ways to proactively immerse their feedback and experience into all an organization does, including something as fundamental as designing a building. For example, Barbara Burke, former vice president and former senior director, Patient-Family Experience at Lurie Children's Hospital of Chicago, as well as former co-leader of The Beryl Institute's Pediatric Community, shared several examples of how the Family & Kids Advisory Board has influenced decisions at Lurie Children's, one of which was the actual design of the hospital's chapel.

The planning team had enlisted a well-known and respected stained-glass company to design traditional chapel windows and was excited about the beautiful new designs, which they proudly brought to the Family & Kids Advisory Board. However, the feedback was not what they had expected. Though the members acknowledged the beauty in the designs, they expressed a concern that they were dark— reminiscent of death and sorrow. They strongly felt that the art just wasn't right for a children's hospital chapel. Listening to their feedback, Lurie's staff partnered with another designer to create art that was more representative of life, with bright colors and simple designs. "It was a watershed moment," Burke explains. "The chapel is now a beautiful, convertible space where people can go to pray and participate in other religious activities."[42]

This example demonstrates the significance of being proactive, not only from an engagement standpoint but also from a financial one. Without this crucial feedback from the outset, the hospital would have invested a large sum of money to create something that those it was intended to serve would not have enjoyed. If they had been reactionary and asked the patients after the fact, it would have not only resulted in a negative experience but also left them in a predicament between leaving it alone or investing even more to demolish the chapel and start over.

What matters most is that an organization finds ways to engage the diverse voices of patients and care partners that are representative of its community through whatever means make the most sense for each of them. A PFAC simply happens to be one of them. Though we believe in the value of PFACs, we are also not arguing that every health organization needs to have one. But if an organization does choose to use a PFAC, it must be intentional about purposely seeking to ensure that it is reflective of the community that the organization serves. One issue that often surfaces with PFACs is that they fail to be demographically reflective of the communities that the healthcare organizations serve. We cannot overlook this reality or its impact on receiving the most representative and effective input.

Outside of PFACs, many other strategies exist to collect quality real-time feedback, including bedside feedback from rounding, app-based feedback, and pulse surveys. With the right infrastructure internally, organizations can also invite patients and care partners to board meetings or ensure that they are represented on various committees so that their stories can be shared, bringing their voices to the top leadership levels. They can institute email programs equipped with survey questions to facilitate continuous feedback loops or utilize E-panels (a prevalent method for collecting diverse perspectives). However, these efforts all must be driven internally. Although we recognize the presence of these methods, what we are talking about in this chapter extends beyond patient satisfaction surveys, as they are just one element within a broader portfolio of tools aimed at engaging diverse voices.

EVOLVING INTO A CO-DESIGNING PARTNERSHIP

Regardless of whether a PFAC or some other means is utilized in partnering and co-designing with patients and care partners, central to any experience strategy are the voices and contributions from those receiving and delivering care as well as the communities that organizations serve. Organizations can be successful without one if they have other strategies for gathering diverse patient and care partner feedback representative of the communities they serve and integrating that feedback as an ongoing process, rather than a recurring project. It is finding out what matters most to the people who matter the most—and then timely doing something about it.

Partnerships with patients and care partners have continued to evolve from the early days of consumer advisory boards in the 1980s to the PFAC model just discussed that took off in the 1990s. Over time, the ways that organizations bring the lived experience of patients and families center stage to healthcare's strategic improvement processes has transformed. Mark Agathangelou, a lived experience partner of NHS England, has provided an example that showcased the role of co-production. A clinical director had developed a questionnaire in consultation with people with lived experience. By checking with a patient group about the wording of the questionnaire, he immediately improved their response rate from 17 percent to 50 percent. "You should be asking people," Mark notes. "It shouldn't be a top-down approach. That is not ethical or democratic."[43]

It is important to affirm from the start that a commitment to engagement is not just a "rubber stamp" from PFAs asked for input after decisions are made. Rather, to be most effective, healthcare organizations should engage patients and care partners as co-creators in a proactive way. Being reactive and asking PFAs what they thought of a decision after the fact or using them as a sounding board misses the mark. Instead, PFAs must be engaged in co-designing the experience that people have— both for themselves in their own individual paths and for others.

How patients and care partners are solicited, valued, and utilized for improvement has nurtured a new perception that healthcare can learn from their experiences. Through all the change, one constant has remained: what differentiates organizations that believe this to be true and those that do not is listening. "Listening organizations" are those that intentionally dispatch staff, meeting people where they are to capture the lived experience of patients, and creatively using innovation and technology to connect with those whom they serve. They heed the advice of patients and families and not only listen to but also act on the opinions of those living the experience, thereby increasing trust and, ultimately, providing better care overall.

As the paper "Listening Organizations: Elevating the Human Experience in Healthcare through the Lived Experience of Patient & Families" notes, "Transitioning from traditional patient and family advisory councils to co-production design teams, organizations are listening to and acting on the lived experience of patients and families, bringing their diverse voices center stage to strategic improvement processes and seeing dramatic results."[44]

There are critical actions that listening organizations take in transforming human experience in healthcare, including the following:

- Asking for feedback with deliberate intention
- Building advisory programs with inclusive and diverse representation
- Seeking out innovation and technology
- Sharing knowledge through structural alignment and collaboration
- Providing patients, their families, and care partners with education training and peer support
- Embracing core concepts of patient- and family-centered care into organizational culture[45]

We again circle back to the premise of listening to the diverse views that represent the communities we serve. These six actions are all founded on communication and trust. They are each about ensuring that patients, family members, and care partners feel that they have a say in the collaboration that inevitably morphs into their experience. Listening organizations incorporate the lived experience of patients and care partners in strategic planning. They have instilled a mindset among all to always improve, deliberately and intentionally asking patients and families what is most important to them. They are dedicated and committed to specific, inclusive actions that fully embed diverse and equitable voices into committees, education, research, and an organization's standard operations.

Perhaps equally as important as listening is communicating what action an organization has taken to address feedback. Cathleen Wheatley, president of Atrium Health Wake Forest Baptist Medical Center in Winston Salem, North Carolina, recalls a time when construction of a new tower required significant changes in parking. Both patients and staff were frustrated. The solution that the organization came up with was to make an investment in golf carts to transport patients, hire people to drive the golf carts, put signage everywhere, and increase communication to patients about the internal wayfinding app via the patient portal. "Every time something comes up," she says, "you have to really listen to your constituents, and you have to let them know you've heard them and what you're doing to make things better for them."

UNDERSTANDING THE ROLE OF CARE PARTNERS

There are an estimated 53 million family care partners in the United States alone. Sixty-one percent are women. Sixty-one percent work. Almost a quarter of them are caring for more than one person.[46] Care partners are undoubtedly a significant extension of the care team. They are not visitors. They are the watchdogs, constantly paying close attention to what is happening around them and looking critically to ensure that their loved one is receiving proper care. They also assist directly in that care and even have a profound impact on safety (discussed ahead).

Still, care partners frequently feel overlooked by healthcare professionals, despite all the immense responsibilities they shoulder in playing this crucial role. "My biggest challenge in interfacing with the healthcare system on behalf of my mom, dad, and sister Karen was the lack of integration and communication among their practitioners," admits former care partner Amy Goyer. "It was entirely up to me to share any updates, medication changes, or treatments with each doctor. Some didn't even seem interested. It was so frustrating and added so much stress to my caregiving journey. I'm happy to advocate for my loved ones, but it would be so much easier to do if the healthcare system would cooperate and collaborate!"[47]

Caregiving encompasses a wide range of roles, from spouses supporting each other during surgeries and treatments to parents caring for children with special needs to close friends advocating for someone who has no one else to do so. Regardless of the specific role, they face significant challenges that often impact their own health, families, and careers. "As a young caregiver, I was 'invisible' for years," notes MaryAnne Sterling, a care partner and patient advocate. "Every major decision I made ... where I lived, my career, my financial well-being ... were all impacted by my caregiving responsibilities. Eventually, my own health suffered because of the stress. Nobody knew."[48]

We must do better. Care partners are critical to positive and successful patient outcomes, and they have their own "caregiver experience" that is distinct from patient experience. They also provide incredible value in frequently identifying gaps in care and services that prevent patients from achieving their goals and function as important voices in decision-making. This all plays out against a backdrop where healthcare organizations across the country are understaffed—and likely will be for many years to come. With care partners present, serving as an advocate for their loved one and even helping to ensure safety, they provide an invaluable service that is, in fact, needed.

Organizations that embrace the care partner experience have established best practices around engaging care partners, including accommodating reasonable visitation and ensuring doctors conduct rounds when care partners are present. Open visitation (as opposed to restricted hours) has been shown to be beneficial for 88 percent of families and has decreased anxiety for 65 percent of patients.[49] Additionally, a study conducted after the COVID-19 pandemic also found that the impact of visitation goes beyond alleviating anxiety and well into safety measures. According to the data, in-hospital fall rates took a significant leap of 100 percent in the months without visitation versus those with no or only some presence allowed.[50]

Globally, there is a significant gap between the perceived notion of what engaging patients and care partners means and the reality of that experience. Though they are often recognized as important, their lived experience is not always fully acknowledged proactively, intentionally, or with the understanding that there are different types of engagement. This approach reflects a unique and underappreciated aspect of patient engagement within healthcare organizations. Connecting with patients and care partners while in the care process helps to ensure an improved experience and better outcomes overall. Simultaneously engaging with others in the overarching healthcare environment helps ensure that an organization is continuously improving. It is the intersection of these intentional engagements and co-design that ultimately enhances and elevates patient experience.

Many organizations attempt to address these critical issues by simply ramping up survey efforts, but this approach overlooks a significant aspect of the process. Relying solely on data collected from a survey simply won't suffice. True progress can only be achieved by complementing that data with active listening in order to understand the often nuanced responses and messages contained therein.

Patients and care partners are not mere helpers or sounding boards; they are valuable advisors and educators for healthcare organizations. They are partners in, and co-designers of, the care process. Their voices possess the potential to drive essential improvements in healthcare for the future. The questions are, "Are we listening? And are we doing anything about it?"

What Is the Impact?

- Strengthened patient partnership
- Improved clinical outcomes
- Increased quality and safety

CHAPTER 7

All Touch Points and Every Interaction Matter

Guiding Principle: Acknowledge that the healthcare experience reaches beyond clinical interactions to all touch points across the continuum of care

Key Takeaways

1. Experience encompasses the entire journey from when a patient first learns about a healthcare organization to well after their clinical encounter.
2. It is important to address the transitions between care settings and non-clinical interactions as critical touch points in someone's overall experience.
3. Proactively anticipating patient needs and addressing potential issues before they arise reduces the need for service recovery and lead to a more positive experience.

"Mind the gap" is a phrase most often associated with the Tube in London. Those three words signal passengers to be cautious of the space between the platform and the train door when boarding or disembarking. It serves as a reminder to watch out for potential hazards or discrepancies that can occur when least expected. Similarly, this well-known phrase helps reframe the overall experience in healthcare. It reminds us to be conscious of the fact that transitioning through the space between two experiences is an experience in and of itself.

Far too many get stuck thinking that experience is what happens from registration to discharge, or only in the clinical setting, but this thought process is both restrictive and risky. Instead, we must think beyond these preconceived notions of experience within certain time and location boundaries. Healthcare experience is boundless; it is expansiveness, the very thing that helps build bridges from the organization and its people to the community and world around them.

Reaching to all touch points on the continuum of care, patient experience begins well before and ends well after clinical interaction. It extends beyond leadership, culture, and the workforce because it is intricately woven into all of them. We can do everything we've discussed in the prior three chapters right, but if we don't "mind the gap" before, during, and after, patients are not likely to have a positive experience.

In this way, the entirety of a patient's journey, from before they choose a healthcare organization to well after their clinical encounter, shapes the stories they share with others. And these stories have a cyclical and exponential impact. The experience that one person has with an organization often begins through the stories shared based on someone else's experience. Then, it is the stories that individual shares with others in the community that will impact other people's decisions. This is the tangible ripple effect of experience.

Take, for example, the manner in which some organizations handle billing and collection processes. Though generally occurring long after clinical involvement, it still directly influences the overall experience of patients. For example, being sent to collections due to a billing error over a nominal amount that was already paid will undoubtedly lead to frustration and dissatisfaction. Everything else could have been executed perfectly to that point, but this action alone will likely end up tainting the entire experience. And when that person shares their story with others, this will be the part they remember most. In this and countless other examples, we see that experiences are found not just in the moments that occur but also in the spaces between those moments, which is where things are prone to fall through the cracks.

In over a decade of doing this work, one organization's clear alignment to the continuity of experience stands out among all the rest. The first moments of our visit at Inova Fair Oaks Hospital in Fairfax, Virginia, set the tone for an insightful exploration of what had led to their patient experience success. Directly off the lobby, at the entrance to the café, we saw something we had yet to see the likes of on any other visit: the "Inova Fair Oaks Hospital Patient Journey." In plain sight was a large, framed sign depicting the key steps of patient experience for patients and families. The journey was based on the facility's shared beliefs and composed of six major milestones, including Planning the Journey, Warm Welcome, Lay of the Land, Itinerary, Daily Activities, and Fond Farewell.[51]

It was evident immediately that this wasn't a mere piece of art; it meant something. Each milestone included the practices and processes at various touch points that supported its success—for all to see. Moreover, this was not the only place we would see it. Copies of the sign were also strategically placed around the facility where patients, family, and staff could consistently be reminded of that journey. This sign represented one of the most transparent and intentional patient experience commitments we have witnessed. In fact, it made such a lasting impression that we still talk about it today, some 10 years later. And even that exemplary model could be extended on both the front and back ends to encompass those spaces before registration and after discharge.

THE SPACE BETWEEN

It would be impossible to cover every touch point in the continuum of care in one chapter. However, there are some prominent examples from the impact point of patients that we include herein. In each, it is apparent that those who took action did so because they could empathize with patients and care partners. They could imagine what it would be like to be in their position at that very moment. Oftentimes, those moments are found in the spaces around increasing access through transitions of care, reducing stress and anxiety with the use of amenities and technology, and changing the stories that are shared with others by going above and beyond their "call of duty" in various respects. Creating a strategy to deliver an effective patient experience considers how to make all parts of it easier and less stressful, while providing increased access to the things that matter most to them.

Easing Transitions with Access and Technology

There is perhaps no greater example of "spaces between" than care transitions. As most people can probably attest, being referred to a specialist from a primary care doctor and then to another facility for lab work is unfortunately often far from seamless. However, imagine a patient leaving the specialist's office with a nurse assuring them that their records have already been sent to their primary doctor. This action and communication would clearly enhance that person's experience significantly.

Such an example would not be difficult to manage. Many times, doctors work within the same system, actually making it far easier for them to pass along critical information than for patients to do so. This is one place where technology's impact on patient experience and the outcomes realized through streamlining and automating processes is invaluable. However, transitions of care don't always resemble a primary/specialist setting. Many patients and care partners find themselves in a difficult transitioning position when returning home after a significant health event, where they are left to manage the complexities of care coordination and transition management without support or access to vital information they need.

Scott Overholt, former chief marketing officer at The White Stone Group, Inc., provided a great example of how this impacts patient experience.[52] He spoke about his dad in Florida, who would tell him after a doctor's appointment that everything was fine. Yet with live monitoring, where the clinicians used their phones to record the patient instructions and then share the recording with patients and care partners, he could access far more detailed information.

"If I could hear the actual recording of the nurse giving patient discharge teaching, I would find out Dad has a couple follow-up appointments in the coming weeks," he says. "He has three new medications, all with different regimens, and he has new dietary restrictions. Once I know this, because I've actually heard his discharge instructions as they were given to him live, I can help hold him accountable, which should result in improved compliance."[53]

Not only do solutions such as this one result in more consistent patient-discharge team performance, but they also give patients and care partners direct access to crucial information that only increases compliance. Scott continues, "If patients are more compliant, they're more likely to heal, and so outcomes improve, which can equate to better patient experience and lasting loyalty."[54]

Relieving Stress and Anxiety

Going to a hospital often induces stress and anxiety among both patients and their care partners. Apprehension about a patient's well-being and the complexity of pending medical procedures is significant in and of itself, but those feelings are often compounded by the unfamiliar surroundings and uncertainty about where to go and when.

Comprehending this unfamiliarity and stress, Jim Smith, department manager, parking and commuter services at Boston Children's Hospital, understood the tremendous impact that parking services can have on patients and families. As such, his team made sure that an attendant was positioned at the garage entrance to let families know where spaces might be available. In the event that someone made it all the way to the top of the parking garage without finding a parking spot, they'd have the option to have their car valeted from there at no charge, saving them from having to drive back to the bottom of the garage to the regular valet area. They did this in anticipation of patients' need to start the experience in a more positive way. As a result, patients were not as stressed going into their appointment or procedure and were more likely to be on time.

Smith didn't stop there, though. Inspired by feedback from patients and family members, he had many great visions to further improve the parking experience, including better signage, more automated pay stations with live assistance nearby from greeters (who could also help with directions), a discharge lounge adjacent to the parking garage, spaces with awnings for assistance vehicles in the main drive, a bridge to connect the hospital and garage, and much more. He saw beyond his title and the specific parameters of his role to make things easier for patients, care partners, and visitors and helped the parking staff understand that their impact goes well beyond collecting parking fees and valeting cars.[55]

Though facility amenities consistently rank low in consumer priorities,[56] what is so striking about this example is that it is not really about valet parking at all. Rather, it's about the crucial role that valet parking can provide in ensuring a seamless care experience. It transcends mere convenience or amenity to reach the heart of the matter: alleviating the stress of a parent with a sick child, a frail patient facing surgery, an adult bringing a parent in for chemo treatments. By reducing stress and facilitating timely appointments, they empower patients to engage more effectively in their care journey.

From an organizational standpoint, the ripple effects of this one act of valeting cars have the power to reverberate through the entire day. As a time-saving measure, it addresses the common issue of individuals arriving late due to a lack of available parking spaces. When they are late, the clinicians run late, backing them up for future procedures, impacting not only their workload but other patients who end up having to wait longer to be seen. Helping get patients to appointments on time has the potential to transform this. It enhances the entire tactical efficiency of operations by ensuring punctuality and minimizing delays. Ultimately, it marks the beginning of a more streamlined and improved experience for all involved.

Once again, the cyclical and ongoing nature of experience is clear. Less stress makes patients better, more informed recipients of knowledge. Having more informed patients, in turn, reduces concern, errors, and delays. Fewer concerns, errors, and delays allow the entire process to stay punctual for others who are having their own experience simultaneously.

Rewriting the Stories Shared

In a 2018 study that explored what really matters to healthcare consumers, we asked people what they did as a result of a positive or negative experience. The results highlighted the powerful ripple effect that experience has. In both instances — positive and negative experiences — the top action that respondents said they would take was to share their experience with others. As such, the question becomes, "How do we ensure that the stories they share are positive?"

Every day, the opportunity exists to improve patient experience in touch points throughout the continuum of care. There are countless instances when professionals go above and beyond to ensure that patients receive the best possible experience. These moments occur in the spaces between clinical interactions, where the human connection takes precedence above all else. It's in these moments that healthcare professionals demonstrate their dedication and compassion — where they transcend clinical duties to make a meaningful difference in the lives of those they serve. In numerous ways, Sentara Healthcare in Norfolk, Virginia, has demonstrated this, creating moments to change not only patient experiences while they are present but also the stories they will share afterward. The following are some specific examples:

- A patient who was very confused and distraught asked for a teddy bear, so a nurse made one out of towels.
- To help alleviate anxiety, team members decorated an autistic patient's room in purple.
- A dying man's family requested he be able to go outside. Team members managed to work through several barriers to make that happen, and he was wheeled outside, where his family surrounded and read to him.
- On multiple occasions, team members have helped patients pull off last-minute ceremonies in the chapel, from weddings to vow renewals and other celebrations.

In another instance, a hospice patient had requested to see her dog. Team members coordinated a visit and while there, her Great Dane climbed into bed with her, prompting someone to remark that the dog was "as big as a horse." That comment persuaded the patient to share that she also owned a horse she would like to see. Sentara nurses and palliative care physicians were listening and developed a plan to allow this medically frail patient to see her horse, Romeo, in the hospital's healing garden. Staff from her stable walked Romeo off a trailer and into the garden, where he laid his head in her lap and nuzzled her hand for apples while her extended family gathered around. Their laughter, tears, and gratitude signaled success.[57]

At the heart of all these instances is the intersection of initiative and empathy— taking an extra step because we can imagine what it would be like to be in that patient's shoes. Another example of this approach was at Centra Health in Lynchburg, Virginia. On a cold winter night when a severe

> *At the heart of all these instances is the intersection of initiative and empathy—taking an extra step because we can imagine what it would be like to be in that patient's shoes.*

snowstorm was blowing in, contracted team members went outside during their downtime to scrape the windshields of cars rather than sit and relax in the warmth of the hospital lobby. "We realize patients and their families are under a lot of stress when they're here," supervisor Jonathan Ramsey acknowledges. "The last thing they need when they are discharged is the added stress of 30 minutes scraping their windows in the cold before they drive home."[58]

This proactive initiative taken by these team members, who voluntarily went above and beyond their duties by scraping windshields before patients departed, was self-motivated. No one told them to do it, but a commitment to improving the experience for hospital visitors had been ingrained in their culture. When we consciously prioritize enhancing the overall experience in the choices we make, we empower team members to follow suit. The hospital staff's choice to enhance the departure process significantly contributed to a more positive and seamless experience for all involved. These become the stories that are shared with others in the community.

Shared stories, in any context, cannot be considered without addressing social media. How we show up in the community and the market overall today must invariably include social media presence, despite some organizations not seeing the need for it. Often the first place that patients and care partners go both to find and share stories, social media directly impacts their own as well as others' experiences.

Sarah Gilstrap, director of Healthcare XM Strategy at Qualtrics, shared the importance of shifting the social media spotlight away from the brand and shining it on the patient. "With the patient as the focus of your social media strategy, the principles and benefits of patient-centered care are realized, and you can see they're being recognized through the voice of your healthcare system or the healthcare provider," she says. "Social media could be used for education to increase knowledge around resources and support available for patients and family members and to better understand the medical condition or a diagnosis. In these and other ways, a thoughtful social media strategy centered around your patient's needs can be used as an avenue to reduce barriers to collaboration."

Social media cannot be ignored; to the contrary, it should be embraced by organizations as a way to meet patients and care partners where they already are. The benefits far outweigh any costs in time or resources as it fosters open communication, promotes transparency, builds trust in an organization's accountability, and demonstrates that an organization values feedback and actively engages with patients.

SERVICE ANTICIPATION VS. SERVICE RECOVERY

Regardless of what "spaces between" we are considering, distinguishing between service anticipation and service recovery is crucial in delivering exceptional patient experiences. Service anticipation reinforces the opportunity we have in creating positive patient experiences by anticipating the needs of patients long before they have the chance to express them. In an ideal world, service recovery, mostly involving the handling of complaints, would be unnecessary because proactive measures would have been taken to avoid complaints. The fact that we have complaints and grievance systems in the first place means that we know we're going to make mistakes. So why not shift the focus to work on a system built on preventing complaints from happening?

The goal of this system should be to minimize errors and prevent complaints altogether by identifying and addressing potential issues beforehand. Though mistakes are inevitable, a proactive approach to service can significantly reduce the need for complaints and thus apologies. Fundamental to this is focusing on preemptive strategies to enhance patient satisfaction and loyalty.

A group from NHS North West in the United Kingdom understood this concept. For years, they had been primarily focused on raising the profile and importance of patient experience, working on the very issue of actively anticipating patients' needs versus always reacting to them. In that effort, one powerful tool they had introduced was Care Cards. These eight simple but powerful cards were discussed between the caregiver and patient for a few minutes, after which the caregiver would ask the patient to prioritize them based on their personal needs. Care Cards supported patients and care partners in exploring how the emotional needs and care preferences of patients could best be captured, monitored, and addressed in real time as part of a quality-led care experience.[59] The process reduced the sense of anxiousness that patients brought to the care setting and ensured a stronger and more proactive approach to addressing a patient's overall experience. It also served as an example of anticipating needs—a "mind the gap" moment.

Even with the best of intentions and anticipation, though, service recovery will still be necessary at times. The key is to make this the exception, not the rule. Timely resolution of issues reassures patients that their concerns are taken seriously.

Houston Methodist understood the importance of this and established patient text messaging to capture real-time feedback. According to Ashleigh Kamencik-Wright, MBA, program director, System Patient Experience, "We send a text to patient and care partners while in the hospital, asking if they have any communication or care concerns. If they say yes, we send a follow-up text asking them to explain the nature of their dissatisfaction. We then let them know that we sent their response to the nurse leaders, triggering a real-time alert. Service recovery is now on the same day rather than after they are discharged and fill out a survey, which could be months later."[60]

These actions exemplify the impact of service recovery when it is handled expediently and appropriately. Their patients' challenges are not only heard but addressed quickly to enhance their experience.

Another successful implementation of service recovery occurred at Tahoe Forest Hospital's Briner Imaging Center after they identified significant delays in breast care appointments, which were directly impacting patient anxiety and satisfaction. They immediately knew that they needed to improve scheduling for routine screenings and reduce turnaround times for diagnostic appointments. Analyzing daily and weekly schedules, they identified opportunities to add procedures and streamline processes. By reworking schedules and adding a second dressing room, they increased appointment availability and improved room turnover, ultimately reducing exam times. These efforts had the following results:

- Decreasing the turnaround time for critical follow-up appointments for patients who needed them most
- Reducing the time it took to access a routine screening appointment
- Decreasing patient complaints around turnaround times from the time of a screening mammogram to getting the diagnostic results[61]

Identifying redundancy, waste, and overlap in their processes drastically improved access to diagnostic care, with reduced wait times for imaging results. This type of action has profound impacts not only on outcomes but also on a patient's experience overall.

As these illustrations demonstrate, when we do things correctly, the ripple effects are not only impactful but also far-reaching. Patient experience is not just about convenience or a certain amenity. It's not only about having certain technology or scraping snow off car windshields. It's also about reducing stress, easing feelings of unrest, and alleviating the uncertainty resulting from a lack of access to information. However, we simply cannot separate hospitality from technology, or care from convenience, in reinforcing the experience continuum.

> *Patient experience is not just about convenience or a certain amenity. It's not only about having certain technology or scraping snow off car windshields. It's also about reducing stress, easing feelings of unrest, and alleviating the uncertainty resulting from a lack of access to information.*

The Experience Framework is the integration of each of these touch points, as well as many others—the culmination of which is the heart of the whole matter and essentially our message in this book. Though we acknowledge that many who engage in healthcare may not choose to be there and that they are identified as patients, they are still people, with stories and purpose, emotions and dreams. This cannot and must not be lost.

Understanding that experience does not begin or end at the doors of a clinical encounter must always be where this conversation starts. Thinking with this broader perspective, we are honoring what's important to the people we serve while, at the same time, creating environments for our workforce to flourish in. As we make the choices to demonstrate that patient experience is paramount throughout each touch point, we are simultaneously reinforcing that our workforce matters because they are the ones delivering on it—the valet attendant matters, the billing person matters, the cafeteria worker matters. In this way, the entirety of patient experience is aligned to the shared understanding of who we choose to be as an organization.

> *Understanding that experience does not begin or end at the doors of a clinical encounter must always be where this conversation starts. Thinking with this broader perspective, we are honoring what's important to the people we serve while, at the same time, creating environments for our workforce to flourish.*

What Is the Impact?

- Improved transitions of care
- Consistent brand experience
- Increased loyalty and market share

CHAPTER 8

Equity and Access
Are Non-negotiable

Guiding Principle: Ensure an active commitment to health equity and access to care

Key Takeaways

1. A commitment to actively eliminating disparities and making high-quality care available to all individuals must be an essential part of any experience strategy.

2. It is crucial to recognize and address both personal biases and systemic barriers to equitable care to ensure excellence in patient care and positive outcomes.

3. Effective communication is essential for equitable care, including consideration of language used and health literacy to ensure that patients understand and can be active partners in their care.

Equity issues and disparities in access have been part of the conversation in healthcare for many years. They are found across the various touch points of the experience continuum, contributing to unequal health outcomes that impact both individuals and communities. Though the attention to these issues may have varied over the years, their importance, and the real impact they have on the experience that people can and should have in healthcare, has not. This reality presents both an individual and systemic issue.

From the individual perspective, we must recognize that our past experiences, perspectives, and implicit biases inadvertently contribute to inequities within healthcare systems, regardless of our awareness of them. Even with the best intentions, our reactions can shape unequal outcomes that have the power to negatively impact patient experience. From a systemic perspective, we must acknowledge the larger issues that have created barriers and perpetuated processes that have limited engagement and access. Though some may have been intentional historically, many are perpetuated now implicitly, and it will take clear and focused work to dismantle the wiring that allows this disparity to continue today. We cannot say that we are striving for excellence in experience unless we are working to ensure that excellence is accessible to all in the communities we serve.

We are called upon to lead courageously with the understanding that we are, first and foremost, human beings caring for human beings. In answering this call, we commit to the following in our "Declaration for Human Experience":[62] acknowledge and dismantle systemic racism and prejudice, tackle disparities, and provide the highest-quality, most equitable care possible. This acknowledgment requires that equity and access, as reflections of how we show up for our communities, are central to the discourse on healthcare experiences. They represent our commitment to care for all—a commitment that cannot and must not be isolated solely in a specific operational department and should instead be intricately woven into every aspect of the experience we provide for all in healthcare.

Open and equal accessibility to healthcare extends far beyond physical reach or racial and ethnic biases—it encompasses economic, linguistic, cultural, and social factors that significantly impact the ability of individuals to obtain, and benefit from, healthcare services. Recognizing and addressing these complexities are essential for maintaining a healthcare environment that is truly inclusive and equitable for all. Though this chapter cannot cover every one of the intricate and numerous aspects of access that impact inequities in healthcare (there are full books on that topic alone), it is important to understand that the issues of equity and access permeate every facet of our healthcare system. The following are only some of the many ways in which others often experience these impacts.

> *Open and equal accessibility to healthcare extends far beyond physical reach or racial and ethnic biases—it encompasses economic, linguistic, cultural, and social factors that significantly impact the ability of individuals to obtain, and benefit from, healthcare services.*

RACE, GENDER, IDENTITY

Personal biases, whether explicit (aware of the bias) or implicit (automatic reactions we have toward other people), can negatively affect our understanding, actions, and decision-making.[63] This can show up in a number of ways, including profiling, disrespectful behavior, withholding options, diverting care, blaming and patronizing others, and racism. The consequences are vast and far-reaching, from denied or limited access to the healthcare services needed most and differences in patient engagement to Black maternal mortality and the undertreatment of pain.[64]

Identifying accessibility around race, gender, age, identity, and other characteristics, though incredibly important, really only scratches the surface of the challenges present. Nikki

Montgomery, former executive director of Madvocator Educational and Healthcare AdvocacyTraining, notes the intricacy
involved: "In real life, patients can embody multiple identities
at once, and providers may hold biases against more than
one of these identities. For example, Black overweight female
patients may experience gender, race, weight, and class bias
all at once."[65] This bias has very real consequences in terms
of how patients access and trust healthcare.

On a podcast fromThe Beryl Institute, Nikki continues:

> On a personal note, as a Black woman who has ex-
> perienced bias in healthcare, I find this to be a par-
> ticularly important conversation about trust too,
> because as I enter the healthcare system, I'm not
> just entering with my knowledge about the dispar-
> ities in care that I should probably expect in the
> healthcare setting. I'm also entering with the stories
> of sisters and cousins and aunts and parents who
> have had negative experiences and experiences of
> harm in healthcare. So I'm bringing with me those
> stories of people I know who have been harmed by
> healthcare in addition to just the data on how my
> own community has interacted with healthcare over
> the ages. And realizing that patients come in with
> that as a form of trauma prevents you from being
> able to immediately start off at ground zero for trust.
> That trauma-informed approach that you can have in
> an individual interaction and also at an institutional
> level to realize that harm has been done and needs
> to be resolved, I think, is so key to issues of trust
> because we cannot assume we're all at the same
> starting point. I know that healthcare providers are
> trusted community partners, but in every commu-
> nity, that same level of trust does not exist, espe-
> cially when harm has occurred.[66]

This reality creates trust differences among populations that are central to the differences in patient experience. If someone cannot trust their provider or healthcare organization, either based on their own or another's perception, they will never have an equitable experience. Without trust, they will never feel as engaged, involved, or valued as someone with trust does. However, when healthcare organizations effectively deal with personal bias and systemic inequity, the opposite holds true: it helps to create more equitable trust, which in turn improves experience.

Uncovering bias and then acting when it is revealed requires the diligent and intentional commitment of healthcare organizations. It also requires a cultural awareness from an organizational standpoint that we need to treat people differently based on their cultural norms—whether they are from a different country, in the deaf or blind community, or in another marginalized population. Jennifer Carron Passon, patient experience officer of BJC HealthCare and member of the Standing Committee on Equity and Inclusion at The Beryl Institute, discusses the importance of personal reflection and the commitment to expanding these efforts throughout the organization: "It starts at the top with the board, president, and CEO and our executive leaders. And it has to be integrated into our mission, vision, and values and our strategic plan."[67] Only through this collective action, including continued education for professionals and organizations to uncover biases, can we move forward toward effective change in providing equitable access to all we serve.

LANGUAGE AND HEALTH LITERACY

Patients have clearly identified that one of the most important aspects of care is providers communicating to them in a way they can understand.[68] At its foundation, this priority is all about access because if we don't even communicate in a way they can understand, we've already dismissed the entire experience strategy. Yet there are hundreds of people speaking different languages in our communities who come into our facilities every day. This, in and of itself, creates issues of inclusion and accessibility. Ultimately, patients cannot access healthcare if they don't understand it.

Geisinger Health System in Pennsylvania addressed this issue to promote health and equity more effectively after observing that 75 percent of their patients were Spanish speaking. With the placement of 700 iPads throughout the healthcare system for video and audio interpretations, as well as Spanish interpreters and dual-role qualified medical interpreters, they provided document translation of medical records, vital documents, HIPAA disclosures, discharge instructions, patient experience documents, and consent forms, as well as Spanish-language voiceovers and captioning.

They wanted to meet the needs of this population by increasing accessibility not only for them but also for all those who speak a language other than English. For example, the mask-wearing during the COVID-19 pandemic rendered lip-reading impossible for the deaf and hard of hearing. As such, Geisinger began closed captioning for communications that impacted them and brought in American Sign Language (ASL) interpreters throughout the organization. These actions allowed for increased access for those who may have otherwise been inadvertently excluded.

AVAILABILITY AND CONVENIENCE

Healthcare practices have long since operated around the convenience of providers rather than the diverse needs of patients. And though we are not suggesting that providers should be available 24/7, there should be some balance in access around their availability. For instance, consider a working single parent who can only access healthcare services for her child after she gets off from work at 6:00 PM. If the doctor's office closes at 5:00 PM every evening, she is effectively excluded from accessing care. This alone highlights a systemic barrier that disproportionately affects individuals with specific circumstances.

The argument could be made that she has choices, which may be true from another person's perspective, but taking such a position often lacks an empathetic recognition of her reality. What are the implications of those choices? Essentially, she would need to take time off from work and likely face financial repercussions for doing so. Further, even after sacrificing part of her workday, she may still encounter lengthy wait times at the doctor's office, exacerbating the strain on her time and resources. The counterargument, then, is, does she really have a *fair* choice?

Susan Pearce, secretary, NSW Health, shares a similar concern noted during the height of the COVID-19 pandemic when isolation was mandated, resulting in disproportionate hardship on certain populations struggling to maintain necessities: "Even with a universal healthcare system like we have [here in New South Wales, Australia], there are groups who we still need to pay particular attention to. We were always focused on vulnerable groups of people because COVID followed lines of disadvantage—people who felt that they needed to go to work because they didn't have sick leave and annual leave and all of those leave entitlements to help keep the roof over their head."

These experiences underscore the inherent discrimination that is often inadvertently embedded within scheduling in and of itself. By prioritizing provider convenience over patient accessibility, healthcare systems have the potential to perpetuate inequities and hinder access to care for marginalized individuals and communities. To more appropriately provide access, organizations can choose to adopt more flexible scheduling policies that consider the realities faced by patients, such as varying work schedules, childcare responsibilities, and financial issues.

COST AND ACCESS

For many, accessing healthcare services is hindered by financial constraints. Affordability is a pivotal factor in determining who can seek necessary medical attention and when they can do so. Exploring the complexities of the financial structure of healthcare systems, which vary greatly from country to country and even region to region, is beyond the purview of this book. However, with regard to the issue of access, it's essential to approach healthcare with sensitivity to the financial realities faced by individuals. To do so requires adopting a patient-centered approach that prioritizes inclusivity and accessibility for all. In this way, we can work toward creating a healthcare system that is not only affordable and, by direct consequence, more accessible but also responsive to the diverse needs of the population it serves.

The impact of inequitable access in healthcare found in these and countless other examples is both physical and emotional, with the loss of trust as a major consequence for both patients and the community—the antithesis of all that we strive to accomplish in providing an exemplary patient experience. "If a patient feels they have been treated unfairly and senses bias is in play, they will walk out and go elsewhere or stop listening and not follow their treatment plan," says Maxine Legall, The Jewish Board's former chief diversity, equity, and inclusion officer. "This will impact how their overall health and lives will look post-encounter."[69]

When we lose trust, health disparities result. Although we are not examining these disparities in detail in this book, our stance remains clear: by approaching equity and access through an experience-oriented lens, these issues are inherently tackled, with trust restored. Following along that same trajectory, a reduction in health disparities would then be realized, fostering more positive outcomes for patients and communities.

MEETING PEOPLE WHERE THEY ARE

Recognizing and respecting the diverse identities and experiences of patients in these ways is crucial for providing inclusive and equitable care. It involves meeting people where they are, both in terms of their healthcare needs and their unique circumstances. However, determining where to meet them requires both a tactical and strategic approach. From the tactical perspective, healthcare organizations need to intentionally ensure that they are hearing the diversity of the communities they serve—that the information they receive is representative of those communities. From the strategic approach, they must commit to taking action in response to those needs.

Tactical Approach: Patient and Family Advisory Councils

As discussed more fully in Chapter 6, PFACs are vital forums for healthcare organizations to gather information. Yet they are often composed of individuals who, while having the capacity to participate, lack representation from the communities that an organization primarily serves. Consequently, their perspectives may be skewed toward certain demographics and not fully reflective of the varied needs and experiences of an organization's full patient population.

Without diverse representation, we risk making decisions based on incomplete information. Not only does this hinder our ability to address the multifaceted needs of the patient population effectively, but it also overlooks crucial insights that may inadvertently reinforce existing inequities within our systems. This lack of representation results in a reality in which our responses are based on partial insights, potentially leading to policies and practices that do not adequately serve all individuals. Jeffrey Cousins, patient- and family-centered care consultant at AdventHealth in Orlando, speaks of this, noting, "Beginning the journey toward diversity requires council leadership to take a hard look at the membership and work to mirror the population served. Consider multiple factors, including race, income, diagnosis, gender, and sexual orientation. Look at the structure of PFAC meetings (time of day, accessibility, etc.) and ask if the structure is inclusive to a wide variety of patients and care partners. If the answer is no, work with healthcare leadership to create a PFAC that enables participation from all the populations served."[70]

Furthermore, many PFAC members serve voluntarily and without compensation, raising concerns about equitable access to participation itself. Affordability barriers, such as transportation costs or the need to juggle multiple jobs, may prevent those from underrepresented communities from engaging fully in PFAC activities, perpetuating disparities in representation, input, and measurements based on incomplete pictures of the realities faced. As such, it's imperative to prioritize gathering comprehensive, representative data that reflects the diverse perspectives and experiences of the communities served.

Kaiser Permanente Northwest did exactly that in working diligently to diversify its pool of Patient Partners and simultaneously make it easier for the staff to bring in the patient voice. Using new recruiting methods, they increased the racial/ethnic diversity of their group of Patient Partners from 5 percent to 25 percent in a three-year timespan, even throughout the COVID-19 pandemic. But that wasn't enough for them.

Their goal was to overcome the barriers to participation. They recognized that traditional ways of onboarding created obstacles to engagement, especially for those who were working parents or for whom transportation to physical meeting spaces was an impediment. They also recognized that onboarding and training patients and families for this role were both extremely important, requiring about 12 to 15 hours to complete, even before the regular monthly meetings. As one way of removing this barrier, they created a new process that allowed individuals to answer surveys and give feedback over email and participate in online listening sessions. For this process, they could onboard new Patient Partners in two to three hours. It also helped engage more diverse patient and family voices because the shortened onboarding process was more accessible to busy people, the surveys and response to email feedback requests could be done at their convenience, and the listening sessions were one-time 1.5–2-hour online meetings.

Addressing these challenges requires a concerted effort to ensure that PFACs are inclusive and representative of the diverse voices within the communities they serve. By prioritizing diversity and actively seeking out perspectives from underrepresented groups, you can foster more equitable decision-making processes and take effective actions that enhance the quality of care you provide to all individuals. These actions will form the foundation of your strategic approach to responding to the diverse needs of the community.

Strategic Approach: A Commitment to Action

Words will never be enough to drive change, but they can motivate us into the action that is needed. Essentially, it's not enough to discuss these issues; we must take action. We must acknowledge that there are things in our way that must be removed or improved upon, which can be as simple as the words we use. For example, understanding the negative impact that a lack of shared definitions and understanding can have on communication, the University of Michigan Health–West created a glossary of core terms to improve the inclusion conversation. These shared definitions strive to limit confusion and division with proactive education. Clearly defining key terms such as "diversity," "equity," and "inclusion" and developing a common understanding around them has enabled those involved to head in the same direction when identifying strategic priorities and initiatives, expedite decision-making, and build greater support for DEI based on what it is—and what it is not.

Organizations that intentionally take action to eliminate barriers to equity and access create a better sense of belonging for both patients and staff. The Beryl Institute's Standing Committee on Equity and Inclusion asks for a Personal Commitment Statement to champion a call to action[71]—once again emphasizing the premise that a commitment without action inevitably falls short. The intention of this statement is to move the conversation on healthcare disparities from ideas to action.

In conjunction with the core statement of "I commit to eliminating disparities in healthcare by driving and demonstrating anti-racism, equity, social justice, inclusion, and belonging for everyone," individuals are encouraged to create a specific action statement on what they are committed to doing by adding, "through taking the following action(s)..." and are prompted with the list of examples below:

- Financially support businesses owned by marginalized individuals/groups
- Honor the differences of others
- Increase participation in organizational and community efforts aimed at eliminating disparities
- Invite someone with a background different from my own to lunch
- Leverage my privilege to give access and opportunities to others
- Make eye contact, smile, and speak to everyone at my place of employment, even those who don't look like me

- Practice curiosity by asking questions
- Speak up if I hear an offensive or discriminatory comment
- Take time to explore and understand my own implicit biases

Though these examples are not all-inclusive, they represent simple actions that culminate in great strides toward removing barriers to equity and access, starting with us. Jolie A. Limon, MD, FAAP, pediatric hospitalist with Southcentral Foundation and former VP of academic affairs and designated institutional official/chief of pediatrics, Valley Children's Hospital, notes, "The time has come when we cannot simply accept the differences we see in health outcomes, point fingers, and blame those who are at a disadvantage. We must look in the mirror and ask what we are doing that allows the system that creates health inequity to continue. It is only when we look inward that we can begin to outwardly move forward to create a health community that recognizes the unique needs and care needed by each human being."[72]

We must move away from the thought that this is about a box to be checked off in a DEI policy. A checklist will not suffice. Forming a DEI department based solely on theoretical ideas of what good should be without an awareness of what is actually happening with leadership, organizational culture, or the workforce, and a clear commitment to action grounded in that knowledge, will not move the needle. Rather, we must understand that this awareness and integrated effort needs to be embedded into everything an organization does to enhance the overall experience, including its impact on the community.

Dennis Pullin, president and CEO of Virtua Health, speaks of the link from an organization to the community in this regard: "We all, as humans, want to feel like we matter, and when we're in a vulnerable position, it matters more to know that someone cares about us, our history, our individual id-iosyncrasies. It really is connecting the organization to the communities that we serve such that there can be a better human experience, and so it is an investment into the fabric of the organization and a part of its DNA, such that we start treating people like they matter, because that's the way we should treat them."[73]

We can list countless strategies, best practices, and case studies, but viewing this through an experience lens is ulti-mately about understanding the far-reaching impacts of eq-uity and access throughout the healthcare continuum. The reality is that these are not separate and distinct from an ex-perience strategy. Efforts to manage costs, service, and care may be siloed off to create infrastructure, but the person ad-dressing health disparities will not be connecting it back to the overall experience if each department remains separate. This is why, with a broader lens of equity and access, expe-rience leaders are the ones who will intentionally determine how to weave all these pieces together.

Similar to the chapters of this book not being individual silos but rather intended to be read together and in conjunc-tion with each other, including their inevitable overlap, so are these issues. Brittany Pope, MS, assistant vice president and former director of applied clinical sciences and research and Institute of Family & Community Impact fellow, OhioGuide-stone, states, "The goal isn't equity in the moment. It's justice, where we won't have to ask these same questions 15 years from now."[74]

When we pull down the lens of our past experiences and current beliefs and perspectives, we can clearly see that each person who walks in the door deserves the same thing. If you believe in human experience, you cannot and must not deny people access to healthcare because of race, identity, ability, etc. When you commit to experience, you are really tightening the seams of all the distinctions in healthcare that otherwise lead to chaos. The closer we can move to this realization and acknowledge that these issues exist, whether we intend them to or not, the quicker we can act to mitigate and ultimately eliminate them—in our organizations and in our communities.

What Is the Impact?

- Reduced barriers to care
- Decreased health disparities
- Improved community trust

CHAPTER 9

Communities Reflect and Inspire Experience Outcomes

Guiding Principle: Expand focus on health outcomes beyond treating illness to addressing the health and well-being of communities

Key Takeaways

1. Healthcare organizations are community based, and the totality of the experience they provide both patients and their workforce shapes the stories that people share.
2. Healthcare organizations must build experience strategy with a clear understanding of the role they play in, and the impact they have on, the communities they serve.
3. Addressing health and well-being at the community level leads to more efficient healthcare delivery, reductions in cost, and a better overall experience.

The traditional approach to healthcare generally focuses on some combination of financial sustainability and improving quality outcomes and overall health. All these factors are, of course, essential; however, in the healthcare world, with an increasing focus on the challenges and opportunities of population health, there is a growing recognition that healthcare needs to extend beyond treating illness into promoting the health and well-being of communities. This shift in focus toward overall health represents a purposeful change from a disease-oriented system to one that proactively prioritizes wellness.

This is an essential component of a focus on human experience overall, as community experience is integral to an overall experience strategy. Healthcare organizations exist in, serve, and are impacted by the communities in which they operate. We can no longer simply think about experience as isolated to the extended boundaries of a healthcare organization or system—experience truly permeates the environments and communities that surround them.

Though some organizations are already addressing this as a part of an experience strategy, it is time for the larger dialogue around experience to expand. The well-being of communities is a natural progression as we seek to ensure the best experience across the continuum of care. Our communities are where patients come from and where they go back to. They are where our own healthcare workforce not only lives but also shares their stories about their experiences.

People don't just accidentally appear at the doors of our clinics, practices, and hospitals. They've likely already heard stories from others about their experiences and are just as likely to tell them about theirs. The perception that once healthcare services are delivered, patient experience concludes fails to acknowledge the ongoing impact and connection of healthcare to communities.

Thinking of the continuum of care as solely within the boundaries of a healthcare organization overlooks a critical context: that these organizations live within communities, not in isolation from them, which requires a different perspective and a broader commitment to action. No business of any kind operates in isolation from its surrounding environment.

In many ways, healthcare may be most influenced by it and has the greatest contributions to make. Communities are impacted by the work that healthcare organizations do. In turn, they significantly impact healthcare organizations. This framing is essential for organizations looking to implement and sustain a successful experience strategy.

In conjunction with this shift in approach is the acknowledgement that the costs associated with a disease-oriented system are pushing healthcare systems to new interventions and alternative models of care. This is based on a shared understanding that keeping people well is much more effective and efficient than healing them once they are ill. It is also grounded in an underlying value in healthcare that is

We have an obligation to care not only for our individual patients but also for the communities that we have the privilege to serve.

rising around the world. We have an obligation to care not only for our individual patients but also for the communities that we have the privilege to serve. To do so, we must expand the focus on health outcomes beyond just treating illness for individual patients and instead promote overall health, wellness, and well-being throughout the community.

If we are to do this, we must shift the paradigm to view "people" and "patients" through a much broader lens when considering patient experience. And through this lens, we can see that experience transcends the confines of healthcare facilities; it's a community endeavor, not merely a facility-based one. The interconnectedness is evident: by prioritizing the health and well-being of the entire community, we inherently improve the outcomes and experiences of individual patients.

The Beryl Institute's "State of Human Experience 2023" study shows a growing recognition of this idea. Notably,

51 percent of our respondents said that they see community experience as extremely important to their overall experience strategy, a figure that jumps to over 90 percent when including those who consider it is somewhat important.[75] Though this is a positive start, we believe that healthcare organizations can and will do more in time to see themselves as even greater parts of the broader community system in which they operate, particularly in response to the social determinants that impact care and the clear issues of equity, access, and continued health disparities—issues that are not distinct from, but rather must be critically integrated into, any experience effort if we are to commit to having a comprehensive experience strategy overall.

IMPACT TO SOCIAL DETERMINANTS, EQUITY, AND ACCESS

A healthcare system primarily focused on treating illness, rather than promoting wellness, will most likely fall short in providing equitable care. As discussed in the previous chapter, such a focus leads to disparities based on factors including access, trust, and affordability, distorting data and obscuring the true impact of healthcare. And merely acknowledging social determinants of health is insufficient, as these disparities are deeply rooted in many of the implicit biases that exist in the healthcare system and perpetuate systemic racism and discrimination. Despite efforts to provide comprehensive care, many individuals are systematically excluded or overlooked—albeit often unintentionally—perpetuating inequities within healthcare. This is why being intentional in building and enacting a community experience strategy becomes so critical.

These social and community challenges, including the realities of health disparities and inequity, all influence how people experience healthcare, so any conversation on human experience must also acknowledge the community and social levels at play. Healthcare's continued struggle to tackle disparities and achieve equity in care isn't confined to any single area; it's a systemic issue that is an illness in and of itself. This systemic illness has resulted in restricted access to healthcare for certain individuals and disparate outcomes for many, especially minority and underserved populations.

Any meaningful change must start with the intentionality and commitment needed to address these problems. When we do more in and for our communities, we ultimately have less to do in the direct care setting. If we create a wellness mindset and well-being strategy that comes from our healthcare systems, we provide better health in our communities. This links us back to the importance of equity, which we addressed in Chapter 8.

This commitment to the overall health and well-being of communities was also explored in the "State of Human Experience 2023" report. In it, we noted that we must expand beyond treating illness to addressing the health and well-being of communities: "Social determinants of health and healthcare disparities must be acknowledged and addressed to ensure a systemic response to care needs and full access to and equity in care delivery."[76]

It is the intangible factors that aren't always associated directly with healthcare that profoundly influence health outcomes. Issues such as food deserts, access to basic screenings, and vaccinations are vital components of community health. Though these factors may not always be directly addressed within traditional healthcare settings, they undeniably impact individuals' well-being and the effectiveness of healthcare interventions.

Alina Moran, referenced in Chapter 5, talks about how Dignity Health California Hospital Medical Center advances social justice by focusing on access and equity in its healthcare system. One of the programs they established helps patients who are experiencing homelessness. Through their Homeless Health Initiative, social workers embedded within their emergency department help patients navigate and connect them to resources. They do this with the understanding that most of these patients are coming to the hospital not necessarily because they need medical services but because of social needs, including a warm bed, food, and shelter. They recognize these visits as opportunities to connect with patients and learn what resources they might need once they leave the hospital. Social workers then support patients in accessing these resources—and in so doing, they are directly impacting not only the individual patient but also the wider community.

Sutter Heath is another organization dedicated to supporting the needs of the community, with a special focus on mental health and support for non-domiciled members of the community. Its emergency department (ED) saw over 100,000 visits per year, among which were 6,733 homeless patients per year and 316 mental health patients per month. Rather than working just to get this population in and out of the ED, Sutter Health staff worked diligently to set patients up to be as safe and cared for as possible after discharge. The ED nurses were careful to explain that some non-domiciled patients prefer living on the street and, with this in mind, they worked to keep them safe rather than try to convince them to change their lifestyle.[77]

If a non-domiciled patient was discharged at night, nurse leaders in the ED would invite them to stay in the waiting room until morning and offer them clean, new clothing and shoes, and even tarps, coats, and other needed supplies, all donated by Sutter Health. Street nurses from Sutter Health also delivered care on the street to ensure that patients were cared for beyond the walls of the hospital. In cooperation with a Sacramento Police task force, the ED case managers helped with services and resources to parents and babies as needed, providing baby cribs to protect against SIDS, food, hotel rooms, car seats, financial consulting, and appointments with a pediatrician for follow up after an emergency visit. The way in which these nurses, leaders, and other care providers spoke about how they helped patients with specific needs and challenging life circumstances was consistently respectful and compassionate.

IMPACT ON THE COST OF CARE

An experience approach that includes the community also acknowledges the impact on the cost of care. Healthcare organizations can no longer support the elevated costs of their communities' health. Evolving over time, it was previously in an organization's best interest for patients to come to the hospital. Now, with overcrowded EDs around the globe and often under-resourced facilities, it's best to create alternative care pathways and solutions that do not require people to present in EDs unless absolutely necessary. This must be part of an overall strategy and has huge consequences. If we can reduce the number of people using an ED for primary care visits, which often strains operations, we can save money within the system, free up critical resources, and provide better care for more people.

Community health centers have also helped alleviate some of this overcrowding, providing accessible and affordable healthcare outside the traditional care settings and pathways and thereby significantly contributing to the solutions we seek. They embody societal, social, and human impacts, demonstrating tangible value to the community. At the same time, by extending healthcare experiences beyond the confines of traditional medical centers and hospitals, these health centers alleviate some of the cost burden on the healthcare system.

More investment in community health initiatives now would yield substantial savings in the future, while greater involvement in communities translates into reduced health-care system utilization, ultimately driving down costs. This alignment follows a simple trajectory: when we improve circumstances outside an organization, we improve circum-stances inside it. With new models based on preventative care, we reduce the extraordinary cost burdens of health-care organizations. This is a direct investment in human ex-perience. When community health improves, there are fewer people who are sick and ultimately need and choose to go to the hospital for care.

In committing to this guiding principle, this is how we must choose to show up in our communities. It is not a marketing or brand initiative. It is not about community relations or hosting health fairs. Though those efforts are commendable, they do not fully reflect a genuine involvement with the community in the way we're talking about. Rather, this is about coming from a preventative, educational, and wellness approach.

Dr. Harish Pillai, group CEO at Metro Pacific Health, notes, "I think it's important that we go back to this whole concept of what the definition of health is. When you put in the WHO definition of health, it talks about a state of physical, mental, spiritual, and social well-being. That is actually what is called 'health.' So we need to look at that kind of a holistic picture because when we talk about social well-being, you need to build [those] kind of conversations with your family, with your friends."

In addition to acknowledging the realities and unique chal-lenges such as these in the American healthcare landscape, it's equally important to draw inspiration from successful models and approaches from around the world. We had the opportu-nity to experience this in our member organizations in Brazil, as an example. Hospital Israelita Albert Einstein established an active and vibrant community health center in one of the biggest favelas in Sao Paolo, where not only was healthcare provided but support for the whole person was offered from childcare and early motherhood workshops to afterschool programs for children and more. Being a beacon for community wellness and well-being must be a central commitment for organizations committed to human experience. This example reflects what many are doing around the world to provide more than healthcare in caring for their communities.

Ultimately, the well-being of the community must remain at the forefront of the conversation surrounding the healthcare experience. It's not just about policies or practices; it's about creating environments where individuals feel valued, supported, and empowered to lead healthier lives. Addressing these complex issues may require a concerted effort and collaboration across various sectors, but it is essential to recognize that improving community health outcomes is within our grasp. It's not a matter of inability but rather a need for deliberate action and purposeful engagement with communities to foster holistic health and well-being.

HOW ORGANIZATIONS ARE TAKING A COMMUNITY-FOCUSED APPROACH

Healthcare organizations are showing up in new, effective ways to address these concerns. The following examples are for illustrative purposes. Though compelling, they are less about the practices themselves and more about the foundation on which those practices are being delivered. They provide tangible representations of the underlying principles and values that inform their delivery. These foundational aspects encompass a range of factors, including but not limited to patient-centered care, equity, access, education, and community engagement. As such, though the specific practices highlighted are significant, more importantly, in and of themselves, they serve as vehicles for understanding and promoting the fundamental tenets of quality, holistic healthcare for the community.

Increasing Access and De-escalation

With the goal of breaking the cycle of patients coming to the hospital as their only means of care, Parkland Health and Hospital System in Dallas, Texas, has embraced the concept of providing primary care services in the community. It has done so in a number of ways. First, the hospital has developed a network of neighborhood-based health centers located throughout the county. These community-oriented primary care (COPC) health centers are located in historically underserved areas of the county.

By shifting patients to a primary care setting once they have stabilized, Parkland is able to provide patients with the services and resources they need while ensuring access to others. Celeste Johnson, DNP, APRN, PMH-CNS, former vice president of nursing for behavioral health, acknowledges that the need is especially great for the indigent population, where fewer in-between services are typically available: "Patients need to be connected to community services so they can break the cycle of utilizing the emergency department for medication refills and non-emergency services that can be offered in an outpatient setting."[78]

Additionally, noting that research shows that responding to a community's growing behavioral health incidences requires more than a police response, Parkland established the Rapid Integrated Group Healthcare Team (RIGHT Care) pilot program. The team consists of mental health social workers, police, and EMS working together to determine the proper treatment for a person in crisis when responding to 911 calls.

On the calls, the team evaluates the situation and determines the best course of action, whether it is an immediate emergency response or a referral to a different provider. On site, the police office screens for safety; the paramedic provides a medical evaluation; and the social worker conducts a psychosocial analysis. The goal of the program is to make sure the city's resources are allocated in a way that helps the most people and handles crises in the field whenever possible. Since the program's inception, thousands of encounters have been conducted. It also offers the added benefit of establishing connections in the community as well as providing analytics for data sharing, answering the long-asked question, "Do they really need to go to the hospital or are there other things we can do to prevent it?"

Preventative Approaches Focusing on Education and Overall Well-Being

In another example from Hospital Israelita Albert Einstein, the organization has long had a steadfast commitment to patient experience. Most critical to this commitment is the idea that "we are never good enough." As we discussed in Chapter 4, a statement such as this is less a self-critique of lack of achievement than a powerful and important realization that in healthcare, when we get complacent because we think we have achieved or attained success, we don't hold that success for long. This idea of constant learning, growing, and acting is not only fundamental to sustaining organizational success but central to the idea that in healthcare today, a commitment to patient experience means we can never truly stop striving to be better.

In one of their many efforts of continuous improvement, those within the organization strive to create personal and fundamental connections with patients, acknowledging them and their care partners as unique in understanding their specific needs. From providing hands-on training for the caregivers of those with dementia in geriatrics to the individual care and concierge services provided in oncology, patients are seen as people with personal stories to tell.

These subtle practices are also emulated in some of the technological aspects of the work at Einstein. As a teaching facility, it provides extensive education and training, including full simulation, not only on the clinical aspects of care but also in bringing in actors who can prepare people for the human elements that those providing care encounter. This represents a powerful commitment to the whole experience, which reaches beyond the walls of Einstein. In these and other ways, they bring their clinical expertise to the far reaches of their community and country, reinforcing their very commitment to social responsibility.

Sentara Princess Anne Hospital (SPAH) also demonstrates their commitment to encouraging well-being for patients and the community in being the first healthcare organization in Virginia to offer the Dean Ornish Program for Reversing Heart Disease. "We felt there was more we could do for our cardiac patients to achieve our Sentara mission to improve health every day," says Dr. Gunadhar Panigrahi, a cardiologist with Sentara Cardiology Specialists. "The Ornish Reversal Program, with its emphasis on exercise, healthy eating, mindfulness, and group support, is an ideal way for patients to be proactive."[79]

The nine-week program is based on more than three decades of research showing that lifestyle changes can treat and reverse the progression of coronary artery disease and other chronic conditions. Groups of 8 to 15 participants convene twice a week at SPAH for four-hour meetings that include one hour each for exercise on monitors, meditation and/or yoga, a lunch, and a learning session featuring nutritional education and group support therapy.

Chris Manetz, director of patient services (cardiology/radiology), talks about the remarkable results of this program: "Since its inception, staff continue to report results in line with the belief that the program can help patients have more energy, less stress, more emotional support, and greater physical endurance. Staff believe that by sticking with the program, participants may reduce their risk of a heart attack, lower their need for medication, and avoid serious interventions such as bypass surgery."[80]

Community-Focused Programs

Bellin Health in Green Bay, Wisconsin, has programs in place to ensure that social determinants of health are understood and addressed for patients. Staff are trained to ask questions about transportation needs, nutrition and food insecurities, and housing. As needs arise, patients are connected to community resources to address underlying situations that may impact their health outcomes. "Many people don't know about support options or they're too ashamed to ask," shares Chris Woleske, EVP, Bellin and Gundersen Health System. "We try to build into our partnership with them that everyone has rough patches in their life. Everybody. You're having a rough patch; that's all. Let us help."

Community-focused programs address specific needs, nurture social cohesion, and empower individuals to create positive change. Spaulding Cape Cod has established a long list of these programs. From a pediatric lecture series to a Parkinson's wellness program, they have found multiple ways to serve patients and families on an ongoing basis. Whether it is wheelchair tennis, hand cycling, adaptive rowing, or windsurfing, those living with disabilities after illness or injury are able to rebuild their strength and sense of independence while increasing body awareness, building self-confidence, learning new life skills, and even making new friends. Spaulding also offers a "Fit to Be Kids" program to encourage healthy lifestyles and weight management for children at risk for health problems due to being overweight.

By providing meeting places for support groups, internships for local students with cognitive disabilities, stroke awareness clinics, preventative screenings, and more, advocacy and community support have been a huge focus at Spaulding. They work with organizations that embrace the opportunity to address community wellness and proactively involve themselves in helping populations reduce the need for care. They have become true partners in healthcare, reaching a new level of patient engagement and experience. Consumer loyalty, brand awareness, and community reputation are all positively influenced by such efforts at ensuring the best in a proactive and positive experience in every encounter.

THE COMMON THREAD

The underlying thread intricately woven through each of these examples is the mindset shift among the individuals within these organizations. Thoughtful, passionate, and visionary leaders and organizations such as these have long since entwined themselves into the communities that surround them. They have established new models of care to make care journeys more accessible, convenient, and seamless through thoughtful interactions with their patients and surrounding communities.

It's essential to weave these examples into the broader conversation about experience. How an organization is perceived and talked about extends far beyond the clinical encounters within its walls. The presence of community health initiatives speaks volumes about an organization's commitment to a system that promotes the overall well-being of everyone the organization touches.

To do this effectively, we must meet people where they are—where they need it most—and then follow them wherever they go, including at home, in their communities, and even virtually. Intentionally considering community well-being requires us to broaden our approach beyond merely treating illness and have a focus that encompasses nurturing the overall health and well-being of entire communities. This entails recognizing and proactively addressing the social determinants of health as well as confronting healthcare disparities head-on. By doing so, we can ensure a comprehensive, systemic response to the diverse care needs within our society, ultimately striving for universal access to quality care and equitable healthcare delivery for all individuals. This fundamental strategy shapes perceptions, utilization patterns, and ultimately, the reputation of healthcare systems. By positioning ourselves as proactive contributors to community health, we not only enhance our standing but also empower individuals to lead healthier, more fulfilling lives.

Our hope is that by this point in the book, you have come to realize that we are not talking about experience in a box. Viewing healthcare through the lens of human experience underscores the importance of reaching people where they are. It's about meeting individuals in their communities, understanding their needs, and addressing those needs proactively. These subtle shifts in approach are pivotal, as they influence the stories told within the very communities that healthcare organizations serve. Positive experiences evoke positive narratives, fostering trust and engagement. As healthcare providers, we face a choice: to sustain reactive systems that fix problems as they arise or to build proactive systems that anticipate and preemptively address issues, promote wellness, and minimize the need for extensive interventions. Choosing the latter will be an integral part of a successful experience strategy moving into the years ahead.

> *As healthcare providers, we face a choice: to sustain reactive systems that fix problems as they arise or to build proactive systems that anticipate and preemptively address issues, promote wellness, and minimize the need for extensive interventions.*

What Is the Impact?

- Reduced cost of care/cost avoidance
- Increased community engagement
- Recognized provider of choice

CHAPTER 10

A Call to Action: The Return on Human Experience

A FOCUS ON OUTCOMES

As we suggested in the Introduction to this book, a strategic commitment to experience brings significant value. You've discovered on the pages since that it also requires a substantial commitment. This commitment to experience excellence cannot be taken for granted—and at the same time, we should be careful not to overcomplicate our efforts. The history that grounds our work and the principles that guide it provide a framework for action and a structure for support to help all achieve success. The ideas shared, the practices presented, and the outcomes suggested all reveal that there is a growing comprehensive and integrated commitment to human experience.

The "how we must take action" was framed around eight guiding principles for experience excellence. These ideas are not standalone silos but carefully linked critical components of an integrated strategy. Our hope is that they will serve as the building blocks for your own efforts. Engaging in the guiding principles not only offers a means to define the kind of experience you seek to provide for patients, your workforce, and your community but also helps you shape the kind of organization you seek to be overall. It comes back to the idea we shared earlier: experience is not just about what you do but is fundamentally grounded in what you choose to be as an organization.

With this perspective in mind, it's crucial to reaffirm that our intent in this book is not to suggest additional tasks to take on. Though we do offer key takeaways and practical insights, it's important to reinforce that what we are suggesting isn't about creating checklists of actions. Rather, we hope you see a strategic possibility that aligns essential commitments with the outcomes you seek to achieve. We hope you see that reframing your definition of organizational identity through the experience you provide is a foundational decision that will shape every aspect of your work and every interaction that people have with your organization.

The key takeaways linked to each guiding principle are intended to provide a succinct encapsulation of the three elements we have seen as essential to effective efforts around it. They serve as a summary of what considerations and steps will help guide you to realize greater value in a commitment to human experience. They reinforce the examples, stories, and quotes presented throughout the book. Designed to serve as strategic guideposts for your effort, linking what to do with why it's important, they stand as a constant reminder of the fundamentals at the heart of experience excellence— fundamentals that you must always build upon as you continue to navigate the evolving experience path.

We are confident that if you wholeheartedly commit to the concepts we've discussed throughout this book, not as something to check off an "experience checklist" but as an unwavering commitment to leading genuine change, your organization's experience will ascend to new heights. And the outcomes you realize will undoubtedly reflect this achievement.

When we commit to this comprehensive approach and ensure that there is a focus on experience in all that we do, the return on investment is clear. Though we have linked specific impacts to each guiding principle, at a higher level, it is a commitment to experience in an integrated way that leads to the greatest impact overall. A focus on experience results in the highest-quality outcomes, stronger consumer loyalty, and the recruitment and retention of the best people for your organization—and it contributes to creating healthier communities. These tangible results all continue to drive value to the bottom line and help ensure strong, financially viable healthcare organizations.

These outcomes are not aspirational ideals. They reflect the realities of what we have seen accomplished in our community over the past nearly 15 years as we have engaged with executives, healthcare workers, consumers, patients and care partners, and community leaders. These accomplishments have all been grounded in one of our founding values at the Institute: collaboration.

A COMMITMENT TO COLLABORATION

We believe that what sets us apart in achieving experience excellence isn't found in individual achievement but more so through a unified dedication to advancing healthcare. It's about a willingness to openly acknowledge our limitations, to humbly seek insights from others, and to freely share knowledge to ensure collective success. We believe that this mindset should permeate every corner of the healthcare landscape.

Collaboration not only was a value that served as a spark when we started the Institute community, but it has also remained essential to our work, reaffirming its importance as the foundational commitment in the "Declaration for Human Experience" itself. As the declaration states, we commit to "collaborate through shared learning within and between organizations, systems, and the broader healthcare continuum to forge a bold new path to a more human-centered, equitable, and effective healthcare system."[81]

This idea of collaboration is not just a nice thing to do— as we shared from the start, rather, it is about driving forward with purpose and intention to outcomes that matter to our community, the broader healthcare ecosystem, and all those who are impacted. It may be a bold goal, but our hope always is that people see experience not just as a task to complete but also as an opportunity to truly transform healthcare. And that opportunity has always stemmed from bringing people together.

We have seen that commitment sprout and continue to spread. With a community of over 65,000 people who have engaged in some capacity as members around the world, and the hundreds of thousands more who have accessed Institute content in almost every country, the thirst for ideas, and also the willingness to share, has prevailed. This has resulted in real and meaningful change. In the "State of Human Experience 2023" study, 75 percent of organizations affirmed that they have a formal mandate for experience. This was the highest level ever recorded since we started asking this question in 2011. This data is about much more than the percentages, though. It represents the story of our community commitment, where we've travelled together on a shared journey of collaboration and transparency, leading us to where the experience movement stands today.[82]

THE VALUE OF HUMAN EXPERIENCE

This commitment is not all that surprising—but it is inspiring. As we've discussed throughout this book, healthcare, at its heart, is first and foremost about human beings caring for human beings. Regardless of a person's status as an executive, staff member, patient, or care partner, we are all human beings with a compassionate understanding of what really matters. And though it may not be exactly the same for every individual, the common desires of being listened to,

> *Healthcare, at its heart, is first and foremost about human beings caring for human beings.*

communicated to in ways we can understand, and treated with dignity and respect bind us together.

In the same way, as we have conveyed throughout the book, if we can build on this foundation of humanity with an integrated and comprehensive approach, we can truly transform human experience in healthcare. That is what the guiding principles help us frame and is what the integrated lenses of the Experience Framework ensure we consider in all the decisions we make in our healthcare organization. It is also why the conversation on human experience itself emerges as so significant.

For almost 15 years, through our spirit of collaboration, we have stood on the premise that we need to broaden our thinking in what was reflected in both the experience conversation and what was possible in terms of the impact we can have. For this reason, we believe, as we remain clearly focused on patient experience, that we must also commit to addressing the reality of human experience that is central to healthcare overall.[83] While we work to ensure that the patient remains at the heart of all we do in healthcare, we must not overlook the experiences of those who show up to serve in healthcare each day or who live in the communities we serve.

We also believe that a comprehensive commitment of this magnitude will lead to significant and integrated results. In our most recent "State of Human Experience 2023" study, when asking people to what extent they believe that their experience efforts have an impact on the following 10 items, their responses were significant, with over 70 percent identifying a commitment to experience as having tangible impact in each:[84]

- Customer service
- Community reputation
- Consumer loyalty
- Clinical outcomes
- Community trust

- Employee engagement and retention
- Workforce trust
- Community health/well-being
- New customer attraction
- Financial outcomes

For this book, as we look deeper at the true return on human experience, asking healthcare leaders, the healthcare workforce, patients, care partners, and healthcare consumers what they see as the greatest benefits of a commitment to experience overall, these three groups reflected overwhelming consensus in the top three benefits that result from a strategic investment in human experience: greater staff engagement and retention/lower turnover, higher patient experience and/or performance scores, and positive clinical outcomes/higher-quality care.

The consistency in the belief that there is real value in a commitment to experience, linked with the tangible financial implications of such outcomes as staff turnover, experience results (especially when tied to reimbursement), and positive clinical outcomes, underlines a clear and compelling case for why a commitment to human experience is not a cost but actually an investment that reaps great benefits and returns. It is incumbent on experience leaders to convey this in all they do to drive positive change. It is imperative that leaders commit to this in action if they wish to realize the outcomes they look to achieve. The value of human experience is realized in a commitment to it, and what we provide in this book can serve as a road map for leaders at all levels to guide the transformation in action and outcomes for their own organizations.

A CALL TO ACTION: WHERE WE GO FROM HERE

Where does this all lead you, the reader, who, through the pages of this book, has begun to feel deep down that perhaps your organization is not providing what you deem to be the best experience? Or those of you who have always been staunch advocates for this work but struggle to get your organization to look at the real value of a commitment to experience and feel the urge to move beyond words on paper to tangible and impactful action? Where do you go from here?

Experience efforts aren't just a list of to-dos but rather strategic investments in the kind of organization you seek to be for all you serve, all who serve, and the communities in which you serve.

We believe that the key to moving forward is found in absorbing and applying the foundational elements we have provided on these pages. We suggest this with the clear reminder that experience efforts aren't just a list of to-dos but rather strategic investments in the kind of organization you seek to be for all you serve, all who serve, and the communities in which you serve. The choice now is how to take the framing offered through these principles and weave them into the kind of organization you seek to run. The opportunity is to engage in the value of a larger global community that surrounds you and is ready to share ideas, practices, and lessons learned, all while it learns from you at the same time.

We urge healthcare leaders to look at experience not simply as tactical but also as strategic and cultural. This broader perspective helps avoid the far-too-common trap of relying solely on tactical solutions. It's not about professional titles, technical expertise, or diagnostic labels. To ensure that healthcare is truly effective and aligns with the needs of patients and care partners, the healthcare workforce, and the community in which you operate, experience must remain central to every intention, choice, and action.

The principles we offer help weave every facet of your organization together. They should not be your next corporate initiative, which has a beginning and, consequently, an ending. A commitment to experience cannot and should not end. Rather, a commitment to experience should embody all you aspire to become. An investment in experience efforts creates a culture shift that has direct bearing on the quality outcomes realized, the patient and family loyalty sought, the community reputation desired, and the vibrant workforce that healthcare leaders strive to ensure every day. And an experience perspective must be infused into every decision, every process, and every interaction you have as an organization.

It is here too that our call to action leads us back to the additional commitments that frame the "Declaration for Human Experience" we shared in opening the book. We can be effective at implementing the suggestions noted in each chapter, but we must remember and step toward these three commitments in all we do in healthcare if we believe in our responsibility to transform human experience. Grounded in the commitment to collaboration and shared learning, we must:

- acknowledge and dismantle systemic racism and prejudice, tackle disparities, and provide the highest-quality, most equitable care possible;
- understand and act on the needs and vulnerabilities of the healthcare workforce to honor their commitment and reaffirm and reenergize their purpose; and
- recognize and maintain a focus on what matters most to patients, their family members, and care partners to ensure unparalleled care and a commitment to health and well-being.[85]

These commitments reflect the very value of human experience itself—that in caring for our patients, workforce, and communities, we can and will significantly transform healthcare. This is no simple effort. It will take work. It will take persistence. It will take resilience. For so many, it already has.

But the results are well worth it and are all that everyone who's engaged in, or impacted by, healthcare truly deserves.

A SENSE OF GRATITUDE

At The Beryl Institute, we have had, and continue to have, the profound privilege of serving as a mirror, reflecting the incredible efforts of so many in our industry. Often, those who are doing the work are unable to fully appreciate their own accomplishments. It is challenging to perceive progress when immersed in the daily efforts and operational tasks of healthcare.

Though we remain authentic and transparent in reflecting this incredible work for all to see, we have refrained from dictating what each specific step should be. We understand and have seen time and time again that what works for one organization may not work for another. Instead, our hope, through this book, is to provide a framework, seasoned with exemplars and samples, that can inspire your own actions.

In many ways, we see our role as that of a catalyst, an agent that provokes or speeds significant change or action. We don't take this responsibility lightly. It has always been our commitment from day one to create a safe space where ideas can be shared and disseminated while inspiring action and change for others. This is the ripple effect that has become a testament to all we do in The Beryl Institute community.

We have spoken throughout the book about the return on a commitment to experience and its impact for an organization, but what moves us toward a better

If every organization were to embrace the real value of an investment in experience and engage in these principles as a road map for action, the result would be transformational for the entire industry on a global scale.

future is considering that impact on a much larger scale. If every organization were to embrace the real value of an investment in experience and engage in these principles as a road map for action, the result would be transformational for the entire industry on a global scale.

The potential of transformation at scale is inspiring. This is the opportunity we saw from the very beginning: that when you bring a group of people together committed to a common purpose in the service of others, profound and incredibly positive things can happen. As catalysts—though our role, by nature, may not be perpetual—it will be through the value of collaboration and a continuous commitment to one another that we know this cause will carry on. For that, we are filled with a boundless sense of gratitude. Ultimately, this transformation will be achieved because of the collective, generous, and significant contributions of so many in the global experience community.

These pages bear witness to the gifts given by this community over the past 15 years. When brilliant, compassionate, and hopeful minds converge to address the challenges and opportunities in transforming healthcare, they generate ripples of hope and possibility throughout the industry. We have been incredibly honored to help foster a space for this spirit of generosity and purpose to thrive.

In the end, our hope with this book is that it serves as a subtle yet significant reminder that if we put experience at the heart of our work, real value is realized—and more so, people's lives are made better in ways that matter to them. That is the power of what this community is and the reality of what each of you does or can still choose to do in transforming human experience in healthcare. For your contributions, commitments, and actions in this community and beyond, and for the impact you will continue to have on the lives of others, we are forever grateful.

Appendix

This appendix provides an overview of Chapters 2 through 9, summarizing the eight guiding principles for experience excellence, the three key takeaways presented in each chapter, and the impact that each of these foundational principles helps organizations achieve, reinforcing the tangible benefits that are realized in prioritizing a commitment to human experience in healthcare.

CHAPTER 2. DEFINING EXPERIENCE IS STEP ONE

Guiding Principle
Develop a formal definition of experience that is understood and shared by all

Key Takeaways
- A clear and shared definition of experience serves as a "true north" in guiding all organizational efforts.
- A definition must reflect the comprehensive and integrated nature of the healthcare experience to inform and guide strategy.
- A definition must be more than words; it is an active and strategic way to engage people in working toward a common purpose.

What Is the Impact?
- Stronger alignment around common purpose
- Increased connection between purpose and action
- Expanded understanding of what experience encompasses

CHAPTER 3. ACCOUNTABLE LEADERSHIP IS ESSENTIAL

Guiding Principle
Identify and support accountable leadership with committed time and focused intent to shape, guide, and execute experience strategy

Key Takeaways
- Experience leaders must have operational accountability and influence and reside in, or have direct access to, the C-suite to ensure alignment and integration with all organizational efforts.
- Experience leaders must be directly engaged in an organization's strategic planning process to ensure that experience is a primary driver of desired outcomes.
- Though experience leadership is a must, the presence of an individual leader does not relieve all members of an organization from the responsibility of delivering a positive experience.

What Is the Impact?
- Elevated strategic commitment to experience
- Integrated approach across an organization
- Expanded accountability for experience goals

CHAPTER 4. CULTURE IS THE FOUNDATION FOR ACTION

Guiding Principle

Establish and reinforce a strong, vibrant, and positive organizational culture

Key Takeaways

- A strong, positive culture is the result of intentional choice and is cultivated through deliberate action and consistent reinforcement.
- The commitment of leadership to model expected behaviors and actions is essential to establishing and sustaining a positive organizational culture.
- A strong organizational culture serves as the foundation from which people make choices and shapes their interactions with others.

What Is the Impact?

- Increased workplace safety
- Sustained high reliability
- Boosted external ratings

CHAPTER 5. PEOPLE ARE THE PRIMARY DRIVERS OF EXPERIENCE

Guiding Principle

Understand and act on the needs and vulnerabilities of the healthcare workforce

Key Takeaways

- The healthcare workforce is the primary conduit through which any experience is delivered.
- Organizations must support and care for their workforce in order to foster engagement, wellness, and growth.
- Active engagement of the healthcare workforce is vital and involves not just listening to their concerns but also taking meaningful actions based on their feedback.

What Is the Impact?

- Improved workforce engagement
- Elevated team member attraction/retention
- Enhanced workforce well-being

CHAPTER 6. ENGAGING PATIENTS AND CARE PARTNERS IS A MUST

Guiding Principle

Implement a defined process for formal, intentional, and continuous partnerships with patients, families, and care partners

Key Takeaways
- Patients and care partners must be intentionally and actively engaged as co-designers in the care process and included as key members of their care team.
- Healthcare organizations must understand and address what matters most to patients and their care partners and ensure that their voices are integral in the decision-making process.
- Formal partnership roles for patients and care partners should be established to ensure active participation in the design and improvement of healthcare services overall.

What Is the Impact?
- Strengthened patient partnership
- Improved clinical outcomes
- Increased quality and safety

CHAPTER 7. ALL TOUCH POINTS AND EVERY INTERACTION MATTER

Guiding Principle

Acknowledge that the healthcare experience reaches beyond clinical interactions to all touch points across the continuum of care

Key Takeaways

- Experience encompasses the entire journey from when a patient first learns about a healthcare organization to well after their clinical encounter.
- It is important to address the transitions between care settings and non-clinical interactions as critical touch points in someone's overall experience.
- Proactively anticipating patient needs and addressing potential issues before they arise reduces the need for service recovery and lead to a more positive experience.

What Is the Impact?

- Improved transitions of care
- Consistent brand experience
- Increased loyalty and market share

CHAPTER 8. EQUITY AND ACCESS ARE NON-NEGOTIABLE

Guiding Principle

Ensure an active commitment to health equity and access to care

Key Takeaways

- A commitment to actively eliminating disparities and making high-quality care available to all individuals must be an essential part of any experience strategy.
- It is crucial to recognize and address both personal biases and systemic barriers to equitable care to ensure excellence in patient care and positive outcomes.
- Effective communication is essential for equitable care, including consideration of language used and health literacy to ensure that patients understand and can be active partners in their care.

What Is the Impact?

- Reduced barriers to care
- Decreased health disparities
- Improved community trust

CHAPTER 9. COMMUNITIES REFLECT AND INSPIRE EXPERIENCE OUTCOMES

Guiding Principle

Expand focus on health outcomes beyond treating illness to addressing the health and well-being of communities

Key Takeaways

- Healthcare organizations are community based, and the totality of the experience they provide both patients and their workforce shapes the stories that people share.
- Healthcare organizations must build experience strategy with a clear understanding of the role they play in, and the impact they have on, the communities they serve.
- Addressing health and well-being at the community level leads to more efficient healthcare delivery, reduction in cost, and a better overall experience.

What Is the Impact?

- Reduced cost of care/cost avoidance
- Increased community engagement
- Recognized provider of choice

Acknowledgments

This book reflects more than just an idea or a set of principles. It represents the insights and inspirations gathered on a long, exciting, and ongoing journey. The ideas we share and actions we suggest were not conjured up in some corner office, but rather they were kindled through the grace, commitment, and contributions of so many who invested their time, energy, and heart to something greater: a shared belief that we can and must work to transform human experience in healthcare.

We are able to bring these words to life and hopefully inspire both personal and collective action due to the support of so many individuals too numerous to thank. For every example we provided on these pages, there were multiple others shared in conferences, papers, articles, and cases that fill the library of resources on which The Beryl Institute continues to grow. The dynamic and generous nature of the Institute community is the true catalyst for change in what healthcare can be.

With that, we want to acknowledge the entirety of The Beryl Institute community. It is your passion and willingness to share your successes and challenges—and your commitment to come together from all parts of the globe to connect, support, and inspire one another—that is the heart of all we set out to build as a community committed to changing the world.

We are grateful to our small but mighty team at The Beryl Institute both for their dedication to support our community and for tirelessly working every day to honor and grow our mission. Each of you brings a unique gift that shapes what is possible in all we do. And to Paul Spiegelman, who not only believed in a dream that we could do more to make healthcare better but also provided the initial support that enabled us to grow an idea into a global movement.

Thank you to the Pithy Wordsmithery team, including Deanna Novak, Devon Pine, and Amelia Forczak, for helping us both navigate this journey and turn decades of experience, along with our collective thoughts into words we hope will move others forward.

To our families who have supported us on this journey, our gratitude can never be fully expressed. A commitment to build a global community and kindle a movement is not a simple task. For us, it has been and will forever be purpose-driven work and an opportunity to leave the world a little better than we found it. Your willingness to stand by, support, and encourage us in every step is the foundation that has made all this possible.

And to you, the reader, who picked up this book for a reason—it may have been curiosity or hope, intention or commitment to something greater. For your support of this effort, we thank you, and for what you will do as a result of what you read, we are forever grateful. Here is to a world that understands and lives the true value of human beings caring for human beings always. One we are excited to create together.

Notes

1. Jason Wolf et al., "Defining Patient Experience," *Patient Experience Journal*, 2014, https://pxjournal.org/journal/vol1/iss1/3/.
2. "Guiding Principles for Experience Excellence," The Beryl Institute, https://theberylinstitute.org/guiding-principles/.
3. Ibid.
4. "Experience Framework," The Beryl Institute, https://theberylinstitute.org/experience-framework/.
5. "A Declaration for Human Experience," TransformHX.org, https://transformhx.org/.
6. "Investing in the Bottom Line: The Value Case for Improving Human Experience in Healthcare," *Patient Experience Journal*, https://pxjournal.org/journal/vol11/iss1/3/.
7. "The State of Human Experience 2023: Affirming the Integrated Nature of Experience in Healthcare Today," The Beryl Institute (2023), https://theberylinstitute.org/product/the-state-of-human-experience-2023-affirming-the-integrated-nature-of-experience-in-healthcare-today/.
8. Ibid.
9. Wolf et al., "Defining Patient Experience."
10. "Department of Veteran Affairs Roadmap to Patient Experience," The Beryl Institute, https://theberylinstitute.org/product/department-of-veteran-affairs-roadmap-to-patient-experience/.
11. Wolf et al., "Defining Patient Experience."
12. Ibid.
13. Jason Wolf et al., "The Human Experience Imperative: Practical insights for executives on organizational strategy, structure and impact," The Beryl Institute, https://theberylinstitute.org/product/the-human-experience-imperative-practical-insights-for-executives-on-organizational-strategy-structure-and-impact-2/.
14. Ibid.
15. "The State of Human Experience 2023," The Beryl Institute.

16. Jason Wolf et al., "The Human Experience Imperative."
17. Ibid.
18. Ibid.
19. Ibid.
20. Ibid.
21. Ibid.
22. Ibid.
23. Ibid.
24. John P. Kotter and James L. Heskett, *Corporate Culture and Performance*, KDP (2011), https://www.amazon.com/Corporate-Culture-Performance-John-Kotter/dp/1451655320.
25. "Owning the Moment: The Journey to Culture Change Across a Large Enterprise," The Beryl Institute, https://theberylinstitute.org/product/owning-the-moment-the-journey-to-culture-change-across-a-large-enterprise/.
26. Ibid.
27. "A Conversation with Jennifer Purdy, Executive Director, Patient Experience at the Veteran's Experience Office," *To Care Is Human* podcast, https://theberylinstitute.org/product/a-conversation-with-jennifer-purdy-executive-director-patient-experience-at-the-veterans-experience-office/.
28. Rick Evans, "Enhancing Staff Engagement and Resiliency by Building a Culture of Respect," The Beryl Institute, https://theberylinstitute.org/product/enhancing-staff-engagement-and-resiliency-by-building-a-culture-of-respect/.
29. "Job Openings and Labor Turnover News Release," Bureau of Labor and Statistics, U.S. Dept. of Labor (May 2024), https://www.bls.gov/news.release/pdf/jolts.pdf.
30. "Nurses are at greater risk than ever as they tackle the pandemic, natural disasters, conflicts and political upheaval," ICN (Sept. 2021), https://www.icn.ch/news/nurses-are-greater-risk-ever-they-tackle-pandemic-natural-disasters-conflicts-and-political.
31. "Caring for the Workforce: Five Strategic Areas to Address Well-Being in Healthcare," The Beryl Institute, https://theberylinstitute.org/product/caring-for-the-workforce-five-strategic-areas-to-address-well-being-in-healthcare-2/.
32. Evans, "Enhancing Staff Engagement and Resiliency by Building a Culture of Respect."

33. Stacy Palmer, "Supporting the Emotional Needs of Staff: The Impact of Schwartz Rounds on Caregiver and Patient Experience," The Beryl Institute (2017), https://theberylinstitute. org/wp-content/uploads/woocommerce_uploads/2022/11/ Supporting-the-Emotional-Needs-of-Staff-The-Impact-of-Schwartz-Rounds-on-Caregiver-and-Patient-Experience--mtqiws.pdf.

34. Genevieve Navar Franklin, "'Soul Snack LIVE!' Restores Staff Spirits," The Beryl Institute, https://theberylinstitute.org/product/ soul-snack-live-restores-staff-spirits/.

35. Ibid.

36. *Powerful Tools for Life and Work*, Oakland, CA: Berrett-Koehler Publishing (2016).

37. "A Declaration for Human Experience," TransformHX.org.

38. Ibid.

39. "Listening Organizations: Elevating the Human Experience in Healthcare through the Lived Experience of Patient & Families," The Beryl Institute, https://theberylinstitute.org/product/ listening-organizations-elevating-the-human-experience-in-healthcare-through-the-lived-experience-of-patient-families/.

40. Barbara Lewis, "Success of Patient and Family Advisory Councils: The Importance of Metrics," National Library of Medicine (2023), https://pubmed.ncbi.nlm.nih.gov/37064819/.

41. "Patient and Family Advisory Councils: Advancing Culturally Effective Patient-Centered Care," The Institute on Assets and Social Policy (2016), https://heller.brandeis.edu/iere/ pdfs/jobs/PFAC.pdf; Karin Johnson Kuhn et al., "The use of patient and family advisory councils to improve patient experience in radiology," Health Care Policy and Quality, 2016;207: 965–970, https://ajronline.org/doi/full/10.2214/ AJR.16.16604#:~:text=Patient%20and%20family%20 advisory%20councils%20(PFACs)%20are%20particularly%20 compelling%20as,CONCLUSION; Anjana Sharma et al., "The impact of patient advisors on healthcare outcomes: A systematic review," BMC Health Services Research, 2017;17:693, https://www.ncbi.nlm.nih.gov/pmc/articles/PMC5651621/.

42. Natalie McKay and Stacy Palmer, "The Power of All: Engaging Individual and Collective Focus to Improve Care Experiences,"

The Beryl Institute, https://theberylinstitute.org/product/
the-power-of-all-engaging-individual-and-collective-focus-to-
improve-care-experiences/.

43. "Listening Organizations: Elevating the Human Experience in
Healthcare through the Lived Experience of Patient & Families."

44. Ibid.

45. Ibid.

46. "Caregiving in the United States 2020," The National
Alliance for Caregiving (NAC) and AARP (May 2020),
https://www.aarp.org/pri/topics/ltss/family-caregiving/
caregiving-in-the-united-states/.

47. "We are not visitors: Working together with family caregivers
and care partners," The Beryl Institute, https://theberylinstitute.
org/wp-content/uploads/2023/05/FamilyExperience_CarePartner_
Guidebook_Jan2022.pdf.

48. Ibid.

49. K Simon et al., "Current practices regarding visitation policies
in critical care units," National Library of Medicine (1997),
https://pubmed.ncbi.nlm.nih.gov/9131200/.

50. "The Influence of COVID-19 Visitation Restrictions on Patient
Experience and Safety Outcomes: A Critical Role for Subjective
Advocates," *Patient Experience Journal* (2021), https://
pxjournal.org/journal/vol8/iss1/5/.

51. Jason Wolf, "The Patient Experience Journey: From Warm
Welcomes to Fond Farewells," The Beryl Institute, https://
theberylinstitute.org/product/the-patient-experience-journey-
from-warm-welcomes-to-fond-farewells/.

52. Virginia Feldman and Scott Overholt, "Care Coordination &
Transitions: How to Use Tools to Avoid the Common Pitfall,"
The Beryl Institute, https://theberylinstitute.org/product/
care-coordination-transitions-how-to-use-tools-to-avoid-the-
common-pitfalls/.

53. Ibid.

54. Ibid.

55. Deanna Frings and Stacy Palmer, "Designing Better
Experiences with Patient and Family Involvement," The Beryl
Institute, https://theberylinstitute.org/product/designing-better-
experiences-with-patient-and-family-involvement/.

56. Jason Wolf, "Consumer Perspectives on Patient Experience 2021," The Beryl Institute, https://theberylinstitute.org/wp-content/uploads/woocommerce_uploads/2022/11/ConsumerPerspectives2021-zwmanl.pdf.

57. Stacey Palmer, "Embracing Unique Cultures and Practices within an Integrated System," The Beryl Institute, https://theberylinstitute.org/product/embracing-unique-cultures-and-practices-within-an-integrated-system/.

58. Stacey Palmer, "Building a System-Wide Commitment to Patient Experience Excellence," The Beryl Institute, https://theberylinstitute.org/product/building-a-system-wide-commitment-to-patient-experience-excellence/.

59. Mandy Wearne and Janet Butterworth, "Care Cards: The Impact of Meaningful Conversation and Understanding Patient Preference," The Beryl Institute, https://theberylinstitute.org/product/care-cards-the-impact-of-meaningful-conversation-and-understanding-patient-preference/.

60. "Capturing Real-Time Feedback through Patient Text Messaging," The Beryl Institute, https://theberylinstitute.org/product/capturing-real-time-feedback-through-patient-text-messaging/.

61. "Briner Imaging Uses Patient Advocacy Data to Improve the Diagnostic Experience," The Beryl Institute, https://theberylinstitute.org/product/briner-imaging-uses-patient-advocacy-data-to-improve-the-diagnostic-experience/.

62. "A Declaration for Human Experience," The Beryl Institute, https://transformhx.org/.

63. Project Implicit website, https://www.projectimplicit.net/.

64. Chloë FitzGerald and Samia Hurst, "Implicit Bias in Healthcare Professionals: A Systematic Review," BMC Med Ethics (2017), https://bmcmedethics.biomedcentral.com/articles/10.1186/s12910-017-0179-8; Rachel Johnson et al., "Patient race/ethnicity and quality of patient–physician communication during medical visits," *Am J Public Health*. 2004;94(12):2084–2090, https://pubmed.ncbi.nlm.nih.gov/15569958/; Bani Saluja and Zenobia Bryant, "How Implicit Bias Contributes to Racial Disparities in Maternal Morbidity and Mortality in the United States," *Journal of Women's Health*, Feb. 2021, 270–273,

https://www.liebertpub.com/doi/full/10.1089/jwh.2020.8874; MD Kogan et al., "Racial disparities in reported prenatal care advice from health care providers," *Am J Public Health,* 1994;84(1):82–8, https://www.ncbi.nlm.nih.gov/pmc/articles/PMC1614898/.

65. "The Impact of Bias on Health Equity and the Human Experience," The Beryl Institute, https://theberylinstitute.org/product/the-impact-of-bias-on-health-equity-and-the-human-experience/.

66. "We have these conversations in our living rooms," The Beryl Institute, https://theberylinstitute.org/product/we-have-these-conversations-in-our-living-rooms/.

67. "The Impact of Bias on Health Equity and the Human Experience," The Beryl Institute.

68. Wolf, "Consumer Perspectives on Patient Experience 2021."

69. "The Impact of Bias on Health Equity and the Human Experience," The Beryl Institute.

70. "Improving the Diversity of Patient Partners," The Beryl Institute, https://theberylinstitute.org/product/improving-the-diversity-of-patient-partners/.

71. "Addressing Systemic Racism and Health Disparities," The Beryl Institute, https://theberylinstitute.org/addressing-systemic-racism-and-health-disparities/.

72. "The Impact of Bias on Health Equity and the Human Experience," The Beryl Institute.

73. "A conversation with Dennis Pullin, President and CEO of Virtua Health," The Beryl Institute, https://theberylinstitute.org/product/the-impact-of-bias-on-health-equity-and-the-human-experience/.

74. "The Impact of Bias on Health Equity and the Human Experience," The Beryl Institute.

75. "The State of Human Experience 2023," The Beryl Institute.

76. Ibid.

77. Tiffany Christensen, "Caring Inclusively: One System's Commitment to Experience and Mental Health for Patients and Employees Alike," The Beryl Institute, https://theberylinstitute.org/product/caring-inclusively-one-systems-commitment-to-experience-and-mental-health-for-patients-and-employees-alike/.

78. Michelle Garrison and Stacey Palmer, "Improving Outcomes and Experience in Behavioral Health through Community

Partnership," The Beryl Institute, https://theberylinstitute.
org/product/improving-outcomes-and-experience-in-
behavioral-health-through-community-partnership/?_
rt=MXwxfHBhcmtsYW5kfDE3MTk5NTc2NDU&_rt_
nonce=c28a8f5745.
79. Palmer, "Embracing Unique Cultures and Practices within an
Integrated System."
80. Ibid.
81. "A Declaration for Human Experience," TransformHX.org.
82. "The State of Human Experience 2023," The Beryl Institute.
83. Jason Wolf, "The State of Patient Experience 2017: A Return to
Purpose," The Beryl Institute (2017), https://theberylinstitute.
org/product/the-state-of-patient-experience-2017-a-return-
to-purpose-2/.
84. "The State of Human Experience 2023," The Beryl Institute.
85. "A Declaration for Human Experience," TransformHX.org.

About the Authors

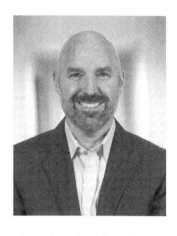

Jason A. Wolf, PhD, CPXP
President & CEO, The Beryl Institute

Jason Wolf is a passionate champion and globally recognized expert on patient experience improvement, organizational culture, and sustaining high performance in healthcare. His driving purpose is unleashing the potential within all of us and elevating the idea that at the heart of healthcare, we are ultimately human beings caring for human beings.

In his almost 15 years as president and CEO of The Beryl Institute, Jason has both grown the organization into the leading global community of practice committed to transforming human experience in healthcare and established the framework for the emerging field of patient experience. The Institute now engages over 60,000 people in more than 85 countries. Jason is also the founding editor of *Patient Experience Journal*, the first open-access, peer-reviewed journal committed to research and practice in patient experience improvement, with readership in over 200 countries and territories.

Jason is a sought-after speaker, provocative commentator, and respected author of numerous publications and academic articles on culture, organizational change, and performance in healthcare, including two books on organizational development in healthcare and over 100 white papers and articles on experience excellence and improvement. A recovering marathoner, Jason sees the journey to transform healthcare perhaps as the greatest race he has ever run. He currently resides in Nashville, Tennessee, with his wife, Beth, and their sons, Samuel and Ian.

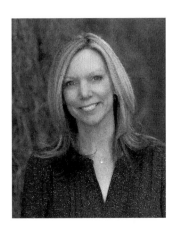

Stacy Palmer, CPXP
SVP & COO, The Beryl Institute

Stacy Palmer is a visionary thinker and pragmatic strategist who has been a critical leader in the rapid expansion of experience as a central conversation in healthcare. Through her role as senior vice president and COO at The Beryl Institute, she has helped expand the focus on experience into a true global movement. With a commitment to gather, understand, and integrate insights from The Beryl Institute community, Stacy helped establish a resource library that shares how healthcare organizations around the world are creating positive experiences for patients, family members, and caregivers. As host of the *To Care Is Human* podcast's PX Marketplace series, she also works with solution providers to broaden industry awareness of the tools available to them to impact experience.

Stacy helps organizations bring experience strategy to life through keynote speeches and workshops. She has co-authored numerous papers and stays connected to the work on the front lines, sharing experience journeys in the Institute's *On the Road* series of articles.

Stacy and her husband, Rick, reside in Colleyville, Texas, where they raised their daughters, Maya and Luca. Driven by her commitment to elevating human experience, Stacy volunteers regularly in the community through religious and service organizations, provides mentorship, and is a passionate advocate for the foster care community.